THE GIFT OF CANCER

LAWRENCE DOOCHIN

The Gift of Cancer

THE GIFT

— OF —

CANCER

**LAWRENCE
DOOCHIN**

With the deepest of love and gratitude, I dedicate this book to God-Great Spirit-Creator, in whom I live and move and have my being. Without you, I am nothing. Without you, this book would not exist. I open my mind and heart to thee so that I can be of the greatest service. Thank you for giving me a life of immense love, joy, and peace. May your Will be my Will.

And I am deeply grateful to my family and close friends who ground me, love me unconditionally, make me laugh, provide a foundation so that I may operate in a difficult world, and who are in holy communion with me at all times. I am so glad we chose to be here together during this momentous time on this planet and I could not do this without you. I love you all so much.

CONTENTS

PREFACE

IF YOU OR A LOVED ONE HAS CANCER, OR ANY MAJOR HEALTH issue, my heart opens to you in the largest way because I know personally how difficult the journey can be. It is really true that one has to walk in another's shoes before they can understand that person's experience.

Not only is the journey with a major health issue difficult, but it can also be very fearful and confusing. Confusion can come from external sources—a wide variety of opinions as to what we should do from others as well as from our doctors—and internally as all of these new emotions and beliefs come up for us to deal with.

One of the major purposes of this book is to help you sort through the confusion, but not in the way you might think, because I don't recommend a detailed path to renewed health in terms of following a specific protocol or undergoing some particular therapy. What I aim to do is to help you to see the areas and false beliefs that are impeding your ability to determine that path for yourself. In order to do this, one of our first starting places is understanding why and how we define others and the world through labels. As we have seen in society, labels can be very misleading and cause great misunderstandings and pain through divisiveness. We want to label ourselves and others as part of some group—liberal or conservative, white or person of color, straight or other, capitalist or socialist, oppressor or victim, religious or atheist, rich or poor—it goes on and on. This desire to be part of a group is understandable because it helps us make sense of the world and because it's part of our DNA from an era when we lived in tribes and relied on group belonging as a survival mechanism.

We label ourselves and others, or we label our experiences and things of the world, to feel safe. But in reality, there are no hard delineations and definitions. These are just constructs we have created. For instance, almost everyone has ancestry that is mixed, many of us have acted as both an oppressor and a victim in our personal relationships, and most of us hold some blend of conservative and liberal values. Labels cannot convey the complexity and individualism of who we are and the world around us. Like a forest, everything blends together and is in a different state of decomposition or growth.

We can't define where one thing starts and stops, and this includes our cancer or other health issues. Our health issues are unique to each of us, and although we have to use some type of descriptor, it is a disservice to say that we are in this particular health bucket or that particular health bucket—especially true with conditions like autoimmune disorders that have a widely varying mix of symptoms—because we start to believe in a bucket with its limited treatment options and limited prognosis. And from there, we'll likely start to take on a specific identity that isn't accurate and which we don't want to take on.

What qualifies as a cancer designation? Is it being picked

up on a CT scan, as was the case with me? Is it showing up in blood work, which never showed up in mine? What size does a tumor have to be before it's called the dreaded "cancer" word? What if no one ever has diagnostics done to provide "evidence" of cancer? There are many people who live with "cancer" all of their lives, and their cancer doesn't grow to create health issues or to cause an early death. At what point do we become a little concerned, moderately concerned, or completely freaked out? Can we acknowledge how arbitrary all of this is?

Of course, cancer is labeled in stages, and there's great fear created when someone is labeled as being in a later stage. But let's first generally acknowledge how this one simple six-letter word creates such fear in us, probably to as great an extent as any other word. The very first thought that a majority of people—and their loved ones—will have when they are told they have cancer is "I am going to die." This is how destructive this word is, and this isn't a good start for our healing journey. But what we need to realize is that cancer cells and precancerous cells are present in everyone's body at all times. When the immune system is functioning properly, these cells are eliminated. So to say that someone now has cancer, whatever stage that might be—as if they didn't have cancer before—is misleading and detrimental to the restoration of good health. You might think this perspective is semantic nitpicking, but as I demonstrate, semantics are an important piece of the puzzle in understanding how we came to our health challenge and how we need to create a broader perspective to achieve optimum health going forward.

My point is that our society uses labels—especially the word "cancer," and even the word "sick"—in a way such that once these words are spoken, they put us in fear and can take away our ability to unemotionally and patiently analyze our situation. Then we have a harder time coming up with a plan of addressing the issue. We have been heavily conditioned by society and a well-meaning medical establishment in a negative way, so we are already in a hole that we have to climb out of before we can even start our journey back to better health. We are really ahead of the game of life if we can recognize the conditioning and realize that life is multifaceted and full of nuances. It's not black and white as most of us want to see it; instead, everything blends to gray.

How is it possible that getting cancer can be a gift? When we speak of healing, what does this actually mean? Most people think it means a complete remission—again, another word that can be misleading—of the cancer, and this may happen. But actually, I mean it in a much broader sense beyond just the physical. We are much more than physical beings. And it's highly likely that our cancer, or other health issues, didn't just come from something related to our physical bodies, like our genetics, or other factors affecting them, like our diets. It's also likely related to our emotions, our mental makeup, and our spiritual connection. This is what I refer to as healing in the complete way. When this occurs, it is a huge gift.

As mentioned above, this book isn't meant to convince you of a certain path to renewed health. As I repeatedly emphasize, each path is highly individualized. But we can't know the proper path for ourselves unless we examine and clear the blockages and false beliefs that are preventing us from accessing our innate knowledge of what is best for us. And most importantly, it's highly likely that these same blockages and false beliefs can be assigned at least partial responsibility for the creation of our health issues. We can't bypass them, or the problem will reappear in the same or a different form. Our bodies and spirits are constantly looking for wholeness and health, to live in a fuller and truer reality of our being.

When we start to uncover our false beliefs, there will be some we don't want to let go of. This is human nature. If something angers you in this book, then it's a pointer to a false belief that you are bumping up against and don't want to take a look at. We only get angry when we are triggered, and we each have different triggers or hot spots that make us angry, defensive, guilty, etc. If it's something we simply disagree with, we move on without a reaction. But clearing what is false within us is one of the primary keys to our healing. We are all here on this earth working to grow in our awareness, and this entails working through false beliefs. Thus, we can take comfort that everyone is in the same boat—although, again, our personal situations are highly individualized. We each have different traumas or conditioning we have experienced that have created our unique belief system, different attachments to things of the world, wide variances in the health of our personal relationships, or whether we see ourselves as a warrior or a victim, for example. Thus, each chapter of this book is organized around a false belief related to the cancer journey that we dive deeply into.

My hope is that my experience with cancer can be a blessing for you. I don't have an agenda here other than your health and joy. I am always wary of someone who has an experience and then transforms it into a large commercial enterprise that claims to offer others the golden ticket—if they do this diet, listen to this seminar, buy this supplement, or do this therapy, among countless other examples. Since we are unique, the one-size-fits-all approach doesn't work. Along with this, we need to understand that our cancer journey isn't something to be viewed as "I need to get through treatment as quickly as possible and have the cancer behind me." Then we miss the gifts. I hope this book will alleviate much of your fear and will clear much of your confusion around your cancer or other health issues, enabling you to see the gifts. As we shall see, our answers and our power lie within us.

FALSE BELIEFS

NUMBER ONE AND TWO

> ❝ *GETTING CANCER IS MY FAULT* ❞

AND

> ❝ *GETTING CANCER HAPPENED RANDOMLY* ❞

THE BELIEF THAT CANCER IS OUR FAULT AND THE BELIEF THAT it happened randomly are two widely divergent statements that I've placed together because they represent opposite sides of the same coin. Thus, we need to explore them together. We humans tend to go to extremes in all aspects of our lives, especially as they relate to our beliefs. For instance, some wealth is not enough—we want to accumulate as much as possible. If we support a certain political party or social group, we assign favorable attributes to everyone who is a member of that party or group and negative attributes to those who are not members of our preferred groups. If we benefit from exercise or from taking a supplement, we believe we should double the amount of exercise or the amount we take of the supplement because logically, more must be better—just look at how the use of marijuana has evolved from its obvious benefits for Parkinson's and other neurological disorders to a perceived panacea for all of our health issues without much long-term research. We want to look for easy and quick fixes and answers, but operating this way doesn't always serve us.

Everything is not black and white, and this nuance holds true for our cancer diagnosis. Whether we're convinced that we're fully at fault or that we're victims of the random whims of the universe regarding our cancer diagnosis, we tend to take an extreme view by blaming either ourselves or others—or God—or we assign no responsibility to ourselves. The truth lies somewhere in the middle. While we are not at fault, we are at least partly responsible. What is the difference?

Fault is almost always associated with blame of some kind, as well as with guilt, especially if it's something we feel that we did and about which we have a lot of regret. But guilt doesn't serve any purpose except to keep us in a state of negativity and victimhood as long as we fail or refuse to recognize that *we are all here making mistakes and doing the best we can.* One of the greatest lessons we can learn in life is self-compassion, and when we have compassion for ourselves, we will automatically have it for others. So what we deem "mistakes" are how we learn to do something differently, since we see that what we did previously didn't turn out to be the best course of action. But what's important is looking at our previous actions or words and taking responsibility without assigning blame, which is badly needed in our world today. When we can take responsibility without blame or guilt, we can clearly see a corrective course of action.

Getting cancer is not your fault, but just as importantly, it didn't happen randomly. Many preeminent quantum physicists such as Carlo Rovelli and David Bohm believe that everything in the universe is relational. Bohm said "The essential feature in quantum interconnectedness is that the whole universe is enfolded in everything, and that each thing is enfolded in the whole." Interaction of all parts of the universe creates the reality we perceive. Certainly, it is also logical that nothing happens without someone making a choice of some kind. If we are hit by another car, we didn't make that choice, but the event happened because the other person chose to be looking at their phone or chose to drive when they did not have enough rest. So, nothing happens randomly and independently of anything else.

Cancer just doesn't show up, even if you have a genetic predisposition to it. Long-term studies on hundreds of thousands of individuals in the UK point to evidence of this. A healthy lifestyle can mitigate a high genetic risk. Conversely, the soaring rates of cancer and other health issues in Japan after the adoption of a Western diet demonstrate the reverse. Our bodies have to provide a favorable terrain for cancer to spread. Our immune system, which is an incredible and complex gift of our humanity, has become clogged and non-functional to an extent where it can't eliminate cancer in the way our bodies are intended to work.

Your health issue, whether cancer or something else, is highly likely to be a combination of choices you have made which weren't aligned with your highest good—the part that's your responsibility—along with choices that were made for you, often without your knowledge or consent. These relate to the world we live in. Again, nothing in the universe is random, since everything is the byproduct of choice—whether it's ours, that of another, such as an individual, group, corporation, or governing authority, or God's plan for this world, if you believe in some type of Creator.

What tips everything over the edge with our health is stress, and when I say stress, most readers will think of a more limited definition. But stress isn't just a consequence of living in unhealthy personal or work situations that give us anxiety. Stress comes from many areas like poor diet, lifestyle choices, environmental factors, unwillingness to work on ourselves and our emotional traumas and blockages, and much more. It is highly likely that several of these factors are coming together to create our health issue—we have just overloaded the immune system to a point where it can no longer be resilient and do its job. We'll look at each of the potential stressors next.

FALSE BELIEF

NUMBER THREE

> **I ONLY NEED CONVENTIONAL TREATMENT**

A S THE LAST CHAPTER TOUCHED ON, OUR HEALTH AND THE development of a diagnosis like cancer isn't random. It comes from an amalgamation of factors that are completely unique for each of us. But what is common to each of us is that we have to eat, and our diet is the most basic building block of our health. Food is a critical energy-giving and nutrient-giving life force for the human body and our existence here, and so it isn't surprising that many studies have shown unequivocally that a poor diet negatively affects our health and is a precursor to cancer and many other illnesses.

Although many still choose to continue eating poorly, most people are aware of diet and health as it relates to eating fast food and junk food. But there is also a lot that is hidden from our awareness. It is important to recognize that we live in a corporatocracy, a society or system that is governed or controlled by corporations. For instance, there is a revolving door of job movement between top USDA officials and executive positions and governing boards for the food related companies which the USDA regulates, and the same holds true for the FDA and

Pharma and for the FCC and telecommunications. The fox is guarding the hen house, so consumers are not being informed and protected. We are eating foods sprayed with acknowledged poisons, genetically modified foods without much or any long-term research on their consequences for our health, meats that are full of hormones and antibiotics—and now mRNA vaccines for pork and beef—foods that have carcinogenic additives and are cooked in cancer-causing oils, foods that are so processed that we receive no nutritional benefit from them, foods such as fish and rice containing high levels of metals like mercury, aluminum, and arsenic, which are also present in many of our household products, foods and drinks that are full of high levels of sodium and of processed sugar, shown to be a major cause of cancer, and more. And the list goes on. Maybe our body can handle one of these in isolation, but it is the cumulative overload that's the straw that breaks the camel's back. One only needs to look at the exponential rise in obesity and chronic illness amongst both children and adults to know that the system is completely broken.

If we were being protected by the USDA, fast food restaurants wouldn't be offering their current fare—even more "respectable" restaurants are also using bad oils—and the grocery shelves would be somewhat bare at this point. Unless we're noticeably gaining weight, which is obviously a big warning signal, we often can't directly see the cumulative effects of eating poorly until one day we are blindsided by a major health issue. And it tastes good, right? So of course, we don't want to give it up to eat that yucky healthy stuff.

In any system, what you input is what you'll get from the output, so no one should be surprised that we will have major health issues if we eat poorly. On this general concept most everyone will agree, but there are widely varying views when we expand to agreeing on which type of diet is best. We are unique individuals with unique genetics, health histories, and needs. There is no diet, no supplement, no prescription medicine, nor any therapy that achieves the same results for everyone, so anyone stating that everyone should be eating a certain way or following a certain health plan is doing a disservice, even though they're likely trying to help others. With everything in life, the middle way and one of moderation is usually the most prudent. But what is obvious is that we need to detox from many things, and this starts with what we eat. As demonstrated through many clinical studies, and especially as demonstrated through rates of obesity, childhood illness, autoimmune diseases, depression, cancer, and much more, the standard western diet is literally slowly killing us—sometimes not so slowly.

If we have cancer, I believe a plant-based diet is critical to jumpstart a detox and give our immune system help. How long that continues is individualistic and needs to be based on what our bodies are telling us.

After eating very poorly—fast food, sodas, chips, ice cream, candy, pizza, and nothing organic—for the first 40 years of my life because I didn't know any better, I transitioned to eating a fairly healthy diet, except for eating out maybe once a week. I ate almost exclusively organic foods with low levels of sugar — though I had some chocolate after dinner—and I began drinking spring water delivered in glass five-gallon jugs as well as water from a filtration system in our house that takes out all of the heavy metals, chlorine, fluoride, and other chemicals. In addition, it also alkalinizes the water, and by extension possibly our bodies, using the natural source of minerals. An alkalized body could be important; some studies have shown that acidic environments help cancer cells grow.

But I still ate a lot of processed chips, even though they were made from organic corn or other non-wheat mixes, and these chips were cooked in unhealthy oils. I also ate a lot of meat with the exception of pork. What was interesting was that well before cancer popped up, my body was telling me to cut significantly back on the meat and chips, and of course, as many of us do, I ignored the signals. It is extremely important to follow what our body is telling us. Unfortunately, in contrast with Eastern beliefs and practices, which value a balance between mind, body, and spirit as well as the heart, Western society highly praises a strong, logical mind. Thus, a large majority of people in the West are not present in their bodies to be able to listen to the signals. This is especially important because fear arises from and is perpetuated by the mind, and we have a great amount of fear to deal with when we face a major health issue.

After my surgery for testicular cancer, which consisted of the removal of my left testes, I had a CT scan which showed that I had an enlarged lymph node in my abdomen which my urologist said was cancerous. This is the area that they would expect to find cancer if it had spread, since your testes start in your abdomen in utero. As we'll explore in more detail later in the book, I waited to determine a course of action. One of the reasons was that I had just been through a difficult surgery— they remove your testes through a large incision in the groin, not the scrotum—and my body needed time to recover if I were to do further treatment. However, I was certain that I needed to make fairly radical changes in my diet, and I was able to pull some good information online related to immune-boosting and cancer-suppressing foods, including roots, herbs, and seeds that are verified in studies. As we have discussed, cancer comes from an overwhelmed immune system, and in order to give an immediate boost to our immune system, we have to first clean ourselves out of as much toxicity as possible through different detox methods, especially our diets.

For about 5 or 6 weeks, I committed to an exclusively vegan diet and consumed no processed foods or sugar. Everything was organic, and I was—and still do on some days—making a delicious smoothie each morning consisting of berries, banana, celery, chard, fresh turmeric and ginger, flaxseed and flaxseed oil, hemp seeds, and other nuts. Sometimes the smoothie was all I felt like having due to the nausea. I was also juicing carrots and still do this intermittently to some extent. After coming across a master Chinese herbalist online who's been treating cancer for many decades, I received tea from him in vacuum packs every 18 days, sometimes with a change in formula, that I was drinking three times a day. Chinese medicine has been treating patients for thousands of years, and we don't take advantage of this knowledge in the West to the extent we should, although the presence and utilization of therapies like acupuncture are growing rapidly. The purpose of the tea was to help with liver detoxification and to boost my immune system in order to eliminate cancer cells in other areas of my body separately from where I was being treated—the herbalist advised me to definitely proceed with conventional treatment of some kind, which I had already decided to opt for.

In addition, I began intermittent fasting, which in studies has been shown to generate cellular and metabolic environments that reduce the ability of cancer cells to survive, helping with any treatment one is doing. Ideally, our food should be consumed within a six- to no more than an eight-hour window between late morning to late afternoon. I found that my body greatly welcomed this change, and I wasn't hungry until later in the morning. Also, it isn't beneficial to be eating evening meals, since this is when our body naturally wants to shut down, following circadian rhythms—the same reason we should be off technology and electronics at night. Circadian rhythms are physical, mental, and behavioral changes that follow a 24-hour cycle following the patterns of the dark and light of night and day. These natural rhythms have been demonstrated to greatly affect our health around sleep, hormone release, eating habits and digestion, and more.

Finally, I used only organic cold-pressed virgin oils such as olive for my salads and coconut and avocado for cooking, since they handle high heat better than olive oil. Most processed products are made with a combination of unhealthy refined seed oils, which have been shown to produce hazardous chemicals and free radicals—a type of unstable molecule that is created during normal cell metabolism and which can affect DNA—when heated, along with a host of other issues, all of which promote cancer growth and other health issues. Because of its low cost, canola oil is used in a vast majority of products but has been shown to be among the leading causes of many modern health issues. But we also have to be aware of sunflower and safflower oils, which are widely used.

Within 10 days of starting my new diet, I felt amazing—I had much more energy, and I was losing excess pounds in a controlled and healthy way. I was giving my body a major blessing and a fighting chance to work on its own as intended. What is interesting is that as we make these changes to improve our diet, our body immediately shifts, and we no longer crave the foods we once ate. In fact, the thought of drinking a soda or eating fast food makes me sick. This doesn't mean that if we love pizza, chips, or ice cream that we can't indulge from time to time, since there are now many excellent healthy and organic alternatives in almost all areas. But you will be surprised how little you crave the old once you make the switch. Your taste buds adjust to what your body needs.

After the initial period, I added back eggs and fish, followed by some chicken, which I had a strong craving for. Our bodies have an innate intelligence, and we need to follow this intuitive guidance. Several weeks later I had a strong craving for red meat, which I honored in that instance and have again when it occasionally pops up. What I did not do was operate based on what others said I *should* or *shouldn't* do. *There is no one size or plan that fits all.* For improved general health, there are those who say we should be on a raw plant-based diet, some who say we should be on an almost exclusively meat-based diet, and everything in between. These diets may have worked for them—or appeared in the short term to work for them—but in no way does that mean it will work for all of us.

There are tremendous resources online for various cancer diet protocols. That is not the purpose or need this book fulfills. Instead, this book is intended to shift your thinking and emotions and to alter your false beliefs around your health challenges so that you can see them in a much broader way in order to find the best path for you as well as to be *free of fear* to at least a large extent.

After our diets, there are equally important factors which have likely contributed to our cancer. Certainly, our lifestyle choices have a major impact. If we use medicators such as alcohol or drugs or tobacco to a large extent, we are adding stress and creating problems for our immune systems. Many individuals are workaholics and their professional and personal lives are not balanced, which also breeds stress.

Our emotional health is critical but usually overlooked. Studies have shown a linkage between cancer patients and extremely low anger scores, suggesting suppression or repression of anger was the precursor to the development of the cancer. These studies also show that repressed anger can be a factor in cancer's progression after diagnosis. It comes as no surprise that trauma we experience has a significant effect in many other areas of our wellbeing. Studies of descendants of Holocaust victims have demonstrated that intergenerational trauma can alter DNA.

I believe in a loving universe that is working *for us*, not against us. In each moment, each encounter, and each relationship, the universe is attempting to show us something that will serve our highest good. We don't want to feel guilty, but we do want to examine our major health issues from all angles to understand possible causes and what responsibility we might have.

The universe operates in a far different and expansive way than we can sense in this three-dimensional world. Developments in quantum physics have given new credence to the powerful Nikola Tesla quote— "If you want to understand the secrets of the universe, think in terms of energy, frequency, and vibration." Regardless of appearances, everything is in vibration and in a constant state of change, even objects that appear stationary. Additionally, many physicists have now come to believe in a unified field. Einstein said, "The Field is the only reality there is," and he used the term "spooky action at a distance," also called "quantum entanglement," the widely accepted phenomenon in which particles such as atoms or electrons have been split and then separated by a great distance. When an action is applied to one, *simultaneously* the other reflects the same action. This is not a book designed to explore these deep topics to any length, but there are several excellent books which do so, including one I recommend—*The Divine Matrix* by Gregg Braden. But the main point for the reader to take away is that there is truly no separation—something the mystics from many religions and spiritual traditions have told us throughout the ages.

Frequency is especially important when we talk about our emotions, because blocked emotions such as repressed anger and grief or unresolved traumas—like abuse or neglect, for example—become energetic blockages in our frequency bodies. Everything in the universe has its own resonant frequency—defined in hertz—from the stars to the earth to the trees and to our hearts and brains and each of our cells. The universe is one large electromagnetic field. Our frequency body underlies and is foundational to our biological body, and distortions in the frequency body show up as health issues in the biological body. This understanding is only in the early stages of exploration by mainstream medicine, but it is growing and becoming more recognized by the general public, especially those in the spiritual community.

We are here on Earth to grow and come to a recognition of a much greater reality beyond this ego-based human existence. The universe presents us with unlimited opportunities and vehicles for us to do this—some "good," like a new relationship or job, and some "bad," like cancer— so that we increase our awareness of our greater selves. The universe is not trying to punish us through "bad" vehicles, but we are a stubborn species, and sometimes we have to go down a harder path because we haven't previously paid attention. We have been tapped on the head several times and haven't course corrected, so something comes up in our life—whether that be cancer, job loss, the breakup of relationships, the loss of wealth—to really make us pay attention. None of us were predestined to get cancer, but the universe uses all situations to help us become more aware and grow. Again, usually the "bad" vehicles arise because we have not paid attention in some way.

As is usually the case, the very vehicle that we are upset about and struggling against and want to distance ourselves from—like our cancer diagnosis, for example—is the exact vehicle that will enable us to rise to a much higher spiritual perspective that we need to facilitate our healing on many levels. Thus, how can we be upset with something that is giving us a gift? We only suffer when we resist and fight against what life is trying to teach us. The very vehicle we want to run away from is the vehicle we need to embrace. So it is really not a "bad" vehicle— we have just applied our judgment system, which is based on our own conditioning and society's conditioning about cancer, and declared it "bad."

Our emotions, like our anger and our fear, are pointers to dysfunctional patterns that we hold and need to release and heal. Every one of us is being pushed by the universe and is working on growth and surrender at different levels according to what is best for us and what we can handle; it is just that some are a lot more aware of this than others. Fear obviously plays a huge role when it comes to a cancer diagnosis, and there is a lot to review there. In fact, I wrote *A Book On Fear: Feeling Safe In A Challenging World*, a book that's really beneficial in helping us understand how to deal with our fears. We will discuss fear more extensively.

If we have been actively working on emotional healing, then we have seen the fruits of our labors in feeling intrinsic joy and peace, being able to move into a space of gratitude with an open and compassionate heart, and especially being able to feel and offer love and forgiveness to ourselves and others. How healthy we are emotionally can play a huge part in whether we get cancer and how well we heal from it. Plato—and many other wise people—said to "know thyself," which means that we must actively explore and face our false beliefs, our projections onto others, our dramas and traumas, and all of the ways in which we hurt others or the earth. A majority of people live unconsciously, often without any understanding of why they do what they do, which can translate into meaningless goals. As we begin to clear these dysfunctional patterns, we not only benefit our physical health, but we also benefit our relationships, our spiritual connections, and especially our levels of joy. True joy can only be derived from discovering our gifts and applying them in service.

Since everything in the universe can be defined in frequency, we can be affected by other's frequencies. Think about how someone who is always negative tends to bring us down. Similarly, our energetics are different if we live in a large city or if we live where we're able to access nature every day. But we also need to pay attention to other frequencies that we interact with every day, like wireless technology. The human body and brain operate at a frequency below 30 hertz, while a cell phone emits a frequency of over 1 billion hertz, similar to putting your head up to a microwave oven which is on and has no shielding. Wireless technology from phones, Wi-Fi, smart meters and more disrupts our normal cell signaling mechanisms and inhibits the ability of our cells to function properly with the clearing of waste and the uptake of proteins—thus making it very difficult for your immune system.

We are surrounded by fields of toxic electromagnetic fields (EMFs), but many of us dismiss a possible effect because we can't see these fields. However, the awareness of this issue is growing rapidly, especially those who have gotten life-threatening illnesses and are courageous enough to look for answers why. The FCC approved 5G, which operates at a vastly different bandwidth from 4G, without any testing—another example of how our regulatory agencies have been captured by industry. There are obviously many other issues with technology, like the brains of children being permanently changed from excessive use, our never being able to move out of our fight-or-flight response conditioning due to constant pinging demanding our attention, our addiction to social media, and much, much more. From gamers wearing diapers to all of the scammers we encounter online, the list is huge. But this book isn't intended to discuss this issue, partially because it's so obvious—it's the elephant in the room that's being ignored. My main purpose here is to point out what—to a highly likely extent—may have contributed to your cancer and other health issues. I am not here to prove anything, and I'm sure that many readers will completely dismiss this, which again is human nature at work. But if you are willing to turn over a few rocks and go far enough down in the search results, you can find a huge amount of info and studies on this very issue. There are thousands of highly reputable scientists, researchers, and health professionals speaking about this issue at the risk of their careers and reputations, and there are significant numbers of studies demonstrating a biological effect from these electromagnetic fields at exposure levels much lower than what we each experience every day. Although I recommend you look for yourself, there are two websites which have very good information you can find in the footnotes of this page.[1]

My cancer was in my left testes, and I would often spend a cumulative hour or two each day sitting in a chair returning emails or scrolling through websites with my right hand and the phone held in my left hand directly over my left testes. While I have no evidence that this direct exposure to toxic EMFs from technology is linked to getting cancer, I believe that it was a factor.

The purpose of this chapter has been, I hope, to broaden our awareness of where cancer can come from and how through our choices, and or through choices made for us—like 5G—we have "participated," however passively, in what has caused our cancer or other illness. We can—and must—look at this reality without guilt. *Any significant health issue like cancer is a major wake-up call.* If we don't recognize the wake-up call and take appropriate action, then we aren't solving the underlying problem. Think of it like having a continual water leak in your house that you continue to clean up without ever fixing the underlying problem from the leaking pipe. We're still offering a favorable terrain for cancer and other health issues to thrive, and even if we are in

---

1   https://www.emfanalysis.com/research/
    https://bioinitiative.org/

"remission," the cancer in our body is likely to return, and we'll have to deal with it again.

Unfortunately, humans want things to be easy, and we rationalize really well in order to fool ourselves. So someone adds some flaxseed to their salad, and they think they're eating healthy, or they give themselves an hour a day off of technology. These things are certainly better than nothing, but they are only a drop in the bucket. Similarly, people want it easy even when they have cancer. This is why so many just opt for conventional treatment, seeing it as the easiest and quickest path. They don't want to make any radical life changes because they're comfortable in their lives, so they think that they're doing something great if they just cut back on fast food or they start walking a couple times a week—both of which, again, are good, since we do need to start somewhere. But we are fooling ourselves when we believe we can make limited changes and that will translate into extreme results. That's not how the universe works in reality. You have to make radical changes to manifest radical results.

I mentioned earlier in this chapter that I ate very poorly until around age 40 because I didn't know any better. As I learned about the importance of diet, I changed what I ate— and my wife and I changed what we fed our children. Our oldest child grew up on a fast-food diet of chicken nuggets and fries, which, she often reminds us, didn't give her the best start. As I learned about wireless technology, I changed how I interacted with it—adjustments like using speakerphone, turning Wi-Fi off at night, keeping my phone away from my body, putting my phone in airplane mode in the car, staying off technology unless doing work or responding to texts, and more. As I gained an understanding of the importance of the emotional and spiritual paths to knowing myself, which happened much earlier in my life, I went through therapy and healed a great deal of trauma and dysfunction, became cognizant of how I often acted like a victim and tried to change that conditioning, vastly improved my relationships with my wife and children, worked on and released my attachment to money as my identity or a defining element of my self-worth, and deepened my relationship with God. The mark of a warrior is what they do with new information—once they know better and can no longer claim ignorant bliss. What will you do with the information in this chapter?

FALSE BELIEF

NUMBER FOUR

> ## I NEED TO TAKE ACTION QUICKLY

MAKING A RUSHED DECISION IS RARELY WISE. THIS PRINCIPLE applies to almost everything in life from our health to our job to our relationships. When it comes to cancer, most people make a rushed decision for several reasons, all of which are based in fear—primarily the fear of death. If we believe in some type of existence after this human-based journey and we have some grounding of faith, we have usually worked at least partially through our fear of death, so our initial cancer diagnosis comes as a shock that temporarily knocks us down. But ideally, we'll be able to get right back up because we're incorporating a higher perspective.

Fear doesn't feel good, and it's a natural human tendency to want to get away from it as soon as possible. But as mentioned earlier, fear is a pointer that can show us what false beliefs we hold that aren't serving our highest good. So, if we sit with our fear and know that it will not overtake us or kill us, we can begin to be okay with it and to look at the false beliefs that are upholding it, which will enable us to make the best decisions for our health—and really everything in life. Unfortunately, in

Western society, as opposed to Eastern societies, we're taught to always be achieving and to keep ourselves busy, so most people don't know how to be still enough to allow themselves to tune into that small, still voice. So, when a physician says, "It's cancer," and says you need treatment immediately—basically inferring you will die if you don't do what they say—we take what we see as the path of least resistance. It's the path of least resistance because we feel that it'll help us escape our fear the quickest, which isn't true, since we aren't identifying the underlying fear—the fear of death. We're therefore not correcting the leak in the pipe. In order to have a complete healing of our cancer or other health issue, we have to fix the pipe.

The reality is that there are only a few instances where immediate action is warranted, and they are usually related to the need for surgery, like if a tumor is causing disruption of blood flow to an organ or something similar, for example. You likely didn't get cancer overnight, and unless it's a super aggressive cancer, it isn't going to spread significantly in the weeks that you need to plan and begin to implement changes in your life as well as to make a decision on treatment. I had a CT scan two weeks after my surgery that revealed that the cancer had spread to a lymph node. My urologist made referrals immediately and said I needed to start treatment—chemo or radiation or both—immediately. I waited six weeks before making a decision to do radiation. In full disclosure, my cancer was a seminoma, which is slower-growing. But if this hadn't been the case, I would have still taken at least several weeks to make a decision. I used this interim time to make physical changes in my life, like my diet and my exposure to EMFs, for example, so that I wouldn't be overwhelmed by doing too many things once I started treatment—although I didn't make the decision to start radiation until at least six weeks post-surgery. I was considering whether I could heal the cancer myself long-term through the changes I was making and through reliance on my faith and spiritual foundation and my understanding of how powerful our beliefs are.

I used this interim period to work through the shock of receiving this diagnosis and the emotions around it. If we're processing an emotional shock properly so that we can healthily integrate it long-term, we're likely going through the five stages of grief as outlined by Elisabeth Kubler Ross: denial, anger, bargaining, depression, and acceptance, in that order. If we short-circuit these because we don't want to go through them (like grief), or we are in fear and make a rushed decision, there will be energetic blockages created as we previously discussed. And these energetic blockages will again prevent us from healing in the complete way. Anything we don't deal with the first time will come back around at some point in the same or another form.

Since I have worked through and processed a large amount of fear in my life—as evidenced in part by my ability to write a book on it—I had an extensive toolbox to apply to the fear, although I actually didn't have that much fear arise. The fear that came up wasn't so much about my possible death, since I am aware of and experience a greater reality than just this human-based one. My fear, however, was related to my family not having me around and the sadness they would experience. I was able to come to a lot of peace about my situation since I knew that I couldn't change it. Peace comes from not resisting what the River of Life is bringing us. Yes, I could have done some things differently, which may have led to my not getting cancer, but this pattern of thought is just meaningless speculation, and I can't change the past. All I can do is make positive changes going forward based on the knowledge I've learned from the past. What we each have in our lives at this very moment is what is, and after processing the emotions around our situation, it doesn't help us in any way to stay in regret, anger, non-acceptance, or victimhood. It doesn't help you, and it doesn't help your family or friends who love you and who are trying to help you through your health issue. This doesn't mean that you don't express when you're tired or overwhelmed—but there is a fine line between asking for help and emotional support and being a victim, and unfortunately much of society these days glorifies victimhood.

What we have been given may be a lemon, but we can truly make lemonade from it. My cancer diagnosis and what I experienced around it was a huge gift and blessing for me. It made me much more present in my body and grateful that I have a body that works pretty well and allows me to experience this life on Earth with a loving wife, children, grandchildren, and friends. I have always worked on centering in the present moment instead of living in the past or the future, and this practice only deepened. If we're exhausted and feeling sick from treatment, we have to live in that very moment just to get by. In that moment we can really see what's important in life— our health and relationships instead of how much money we make or what our career accomplishments are. I surrendered to whatever the outcome would be, and this strengthened an already deep relationship with God and brought me a lot of peace, too. Realizing we have a limited time on this earth can be great manna to push us into recognition of a greater self beyond this human existence—or it can work the opposite way if someone stays in fear. And I became much more compassionate towards others, especially once I started treatment and saw that so many are in the same boat, a trend which, unfortunately, is increasing. I could see the fear in the faces of people who had cancer, and I wanted to just comfort them with the assurance that everything would be okay, one way or another.

If we rush into treatment in order to escape the fear we feel, we will miss all of these gifts. We have cancer either way, so we might as well come to peace with it and see what gifts it can offer. And if we rush into treatment and we never make the changes discussed in the previous chapter, we think we've alleviated our fear, but we haven't, because we haven't given a chance at healing our best shot. We will always have a fear in the back of our minds that we could have done more and that the cancer will come back. This isn't living, even if it appears that our cancer is gone. In this case, we have actually died while we're still alive. If you take one thing away from this book, I hope it is that you can live a love- and joy-filled life until your last breath, even if you are dealing with a severe health issue.

FALSE BELIEF

NUMBER FIVE

I SHOULD DO EVERYTHING MY DOCTOR SAYS

D ID WE DO EVERYTHING OUR PARENTS ALWAYS SAID TO DO, OR do we always do what our partners tell us now to do? Do we automatically do what we're told by the government or others in positions of authority, like a job supervisor? If we automatically accept what they tell us, do we start to believe and take their belief systems in as our own? Will this only take us farther away from knowing what we believe and who we truly are?

We can't separate anything in life, and this reality is especially true with psychology, our false beliefs, and the willingness of a majority of people to give their power away. We do this with politics to a great extent, since we want someone to take care of us. We want to put politicians and people in positions of authority on a pedestal—and we put many others, like celebrities, on a pedestal, as if they have something we want. We tell ourselves that our leaders in industry and our politicians know more than us and we assume, almost always very wrongly, that they will put the interests of others above or at least to an equal extent to their own, especially if they've been elected to positions of power.

But this is not how a lot of humans operate; many are in it for themselves. While many parents may not place their interests above our own, our parents carry their own traumas, fears, and conditioning, which they pass on to us.

So why do we place others on a pedestal and give them our power? What I have observed is that each human has an extremely varied psychological makeup that comes partly from their experiences and also partly from their genetics. A friend of mine pointed out a study done at Stanford several years back that demonstrated that a certain percentage of the population doesn't have the makeup in their DNA to rise above herd mentality, which was eye-opening for me and helped me operate from a space of greater compassion. For whatever reason—whether it be fear, conditioning, genetics, belief in the goodness of man, or something else entirely—some people will automatically give their power away and defer to what they're being told or automatically accept what someone thinks of them. But this way of operating in the world is dangerous. We can see the dangers play out in the myriad historical atrocities committed by unstable leaders all the way down to our individual personal relationships, which can be fraught with emotional, mental, and physical abuse.

I have no doubt that most physicians and health professionals enter the field of medicine to help people, but we need to recognize, too, that each of these individuals has their own traumas, false beliefs, and conditioning. They have been trained in a medical paradigm that is heavily oriented to pharmaceuticals—only one-third of the country's medical schools even teach a course on nutrition. Thus, your oncologist has been heavily conditioned in a certain model of treatment to the detriment of the incorporation or consideration of other treatment modalities to boost the immune system. I have heard numerous times over the years about others' experiences with cancer and how the oncologist will tell patients to eat whatever they can keep down. There is logic to this guidance, but there's also a lot of illogic if the recommended diet consists of foods that are cancer-promoting.

Our doctors are giving us one path among many, and it's important that we take the information in while holding this realization. Other individuals are not in your body, and so they can't feel what your body needs. Physicians are giving a standard recommendation—slightly modified, but not by much—to everyone they see. This is what they've been trained in and are paid to do, and as they should, they will err on the side of caution. My urologist recommended that I do chemo over radiation, even though I was a really good candidate for proton radiation therapy, which is more targeted and less invasive. He was concerned about getting rid of the cancer this time around, but one of the reasons I waited to decide on my course of treatment was that undergoing chemo or radiation increases your chances for the recurrence of cancer in other areas, since you're altering DNA in healthy cells that are more likely to mutate into cancer. I was looking at the long-term, not just the short-term, and I felt good about the proton therapy being much less invasive.

Too many people immediately give their power away and do exactly as their doctor recommends. I understand and have compassion for this approach, but we almost always have to wait and work through our emotions and gather much more info. We need to make a decision from both our heart and our mind. When I had a consultation with the radiation oncologist, he told me that many people never make it to them because they first have a consultation with a chemo oncologist and sign up immediately for that treatment—when it's actually highly likely they can do a much less invasive course of treatment with the proton radiation, which is great for contained cancers such as the type that was in my lymph node, and cancer of the prostate, breast, neck, and other types, for example. Just because some patients happened to visit with the chemo oncologist first and followed their recommendation, they may have taken a course of action with more immediate and long-term side effects. The chemo oncologist is not likely going to tell a prospective client that they shouldn't do chemo and should do proton radiation, since they obviously believe in what they're doing and are usually employed by large corporations—where, of course, revenue comes into play. And chemotherapy drugs are among the most profitable drugs for the pharmaceutical industry.

The above not only applies to physicians treating cancer conventionally, but it also applies to alternative physicians who are treating cancer. They have their own unique belief systems as well. They see health and disease in a certain way and are guided by their own perspectives when making recommendations, some of which might be good for you and some of which may not be. It just so happened that my internist, who really cares about his patients, treats a lot of cancer with diet, herbs and IV therapy. I did a consultation with him, but I didn't follow his recommendations because they were somewhat different from what I had found online and was already doing, and because you can certainly do too much. There is a fine balance between doing enough and doing something to an extreme extent because you're fearful of dying. I felt good about what I was doing, since it covered a lot of areas. And then I let it go and knew that it was in God's hands.

All of these factors I've written about in this chapter need to come into our awareness as we make a decision *that is best for us. This is not a decision that can be outsourced.* You have to make it, and in doing so, you will discover incredible gifts that come from your health issues and strengths you didn't know you had. And you will retain your power and feel good about your place in the great scheme of things, regardless of whether your health issue is eventually what you pass away from. Again, this can be called healing in the complete way.

FALSE BELIEFS

NUMBER SIX AND SEVEN

> ## *I CAN DO THIS BY MYSELF*

AND

> ## *I NEED TO TELL EVERYONE*

JUST AS WITH FALSE BELIEFS NUMBER ONE AND TWO, I'M STATING the two extremes of the same spectrum here, since many default to one extreme or the other. It's important to review that we each see the world through our own colored lenses which are based on our conditioning—how our parents raised us, what we've taken on and believed from society, and what a spouse or supervisor says about us, among other examples. But our conditioning and beliefs are relative, not absolute. If we want to grow, we have to drop what is false to find what is true within us.

We may have been conditioned and taught by our fathers that we shouldn't show emotion and should act strong in all situations. Or we may have been conditioned by our mothers, maybe only implicitly, that we should tell everyone our business, since we want people to feel sorry for us, and that's how we get attention—pity through victimhood. Can we see how any conditioning will create a belief system that can and will affect how we deal with a significant health issue such as cancer—and really all of the decisions we make in life?

As we examine and release our beliefs, we always move towards the middle, towards a place of balance. From this place we will know who to tell about our diagnosis and who not to tell. And this may change in the moment as we encounter situations where we feel led to tell a stranger about our diagnosis. Soon after my surgery, I was talking to a business acquaintance, and I asked her how she was doing. She said that she was concerned about her sister who was dealing with stage 4 cancer and had been fighting it for a year. This woman was not someone I would have normally told of my health issue—nor would she have normally mentioned something like this about her sister—but I knew that life had placed the two of us together in that moment and that I could share some info about diet and other factors that could help her sister. *We are all here helping each other.* But we have to pay close attention and follow our intuition and heart to know when we are supposed to say something.

The electromagnetic field of the heart is 60 times greater than that of the brain, which indicates that the heart field is an extremely active area central to our consciousness and operation in life. How do we access our intuition and heart, especially in our Western world that's so heavily dominated by the mind? We have to practice this method of connecting with our true self. It is actually innate to us, but we've closed down these pathways in lieu of excessive reliance on a strong and logical mind. We can reawaken this access by removing ourselves from the world for periods of time. We can put down our tech and turn off the news. We can go sit in nature away from others. We can meditate. We can engage in practices which take us out of the monkey mind, practices like yoga, painting, dance, or writing—anything where we lose track of time and are present in the moment. We can be grateful—the gratitude we feel flowing through our heart and every part of our being. We can and must ask the universe—what many of us call God—for help. There are also some organizations like the HeartMath Institute which offer simple exercises to start building out these dormant pathways. We want to access these extremely important parts of ourselves; this will have transformative results in all areas of our life, not just our health decisions.

If we reflect back on the title of this section, we can see that our path is almost certainly in the middle between the two statements. It is true that some of us are much stronger than others, but many of us are not psychologically ready to do a proper evaluation of ourselves—to hearken back to that "know thyself" that some pretty wise people have told us. So, it's probably not a good idea to think we are superhuman and don't need anyone's help, since we may be fooling ourselves and turning away emotional or other support *due to shame, guilt, or the feeling that we're inconveniencing someone if we ask for help.* Exploring the reasons behind our unwillingness to accept help will teach us a lot about our false beliefs. We are one human community on Earth, and we are in a multitude of overlapping relationships because they are vehicles for growth and because *we all desire to be in community.* Being in community is part of our DNA, and only in the last 75 to 100 years has this sense of community been badly eroded by modern society—versus the relative eons we have lived in community. So, at a minimum, letting close family members and friends know about your cancer and treatment is super important, but we don't need to attempt to elicit sympathy by acting like a victim. When I was asked, I would simply share with my wife or others that I was very tired or nauseated if that was the case. We all want sympathy, and we all fall into victimhood at times, but we can't stay in victimhood, since that is antithetical to our ability to heal.

As opposed to telling no one or very few people about our cancer, the opposite can be equally detrimental if people are thinking of us as damaged or less than. What science has taught us about energetics is that our thoughts create our reality. In the well-known double-slit experiment in quantum physics, the experimenter shines a light on a barrier with two narrow slits and then observes the interference pattern it creates on a screen. Light simultaneously has two natures: it is both wavelike and also particle-like. What the double slit experiment has demonstrated is that light only becomes one state or the other *through observation or non-observation.*

What is obvious is that what *we think, or don't think,* about our cancer diagnosis and our prognosis is first and foremost the key to our healing. Hope and optimism have transformative effects on healing. But hope and optimism have to be balanced with reality. If we have stage 4 cancer and we think we can pray it away without doing any type of treatment or changing any habits or circumstances in our lives, we're operating from a state of denial—that is, unless we have the consciousness of a highly spiritual master, which is always possible but not very likely. Hope and optimism are innate to us, but they are also fostered when we gather as much information as possible through research and through a course of action, which is an exercise in keeping our power. Information is power. So again, we mustn't blindly give our power away and automatically do what the doctor tells us and nothing else. My hope and optimism started with my relationship with God but were bolstered by understanding what type of cancer I had *and* by taking a multifaceted approach to its treatment. It was kind of like throwing the kitchen sink at it but in an organized and well-thought-out fashion.

After we examine our own beliefs, it's important to understand the possible belief systems and energetics of those we choose to inform about our cancer. Spiritual masters like Jesus and others were able to achieve results based on two factors: the unity consciousness of the spiritual master delivering the healing—knowing what they asked for would be granted—and the consciousness of the one receiving the healing—namely the acceptance that "miracles" can happen in the universe, what many call the Kingdom of God. Obviously, this acceptance is first predicated on our knowing that the Kingdom of God exists.

The power of prayer is immense and should be utilized to the fullest. If we tell a large number of people about our cancer and we even have a prayer chain, how are these individuals praying for us and thinking of us? We need to ask for a certain kind of prayer, since it's likely that many are praying for us to be healed, inferring that we are sick. *You are not sick*, since you are not separate from anything else in the universe, as we discussed earlier. Thus, you are whole but having a temporary health issue that needs addressing. This view is one of fine nuance but also a critical one. The way the universe works is that if someone is praying for you and sees you as sick, they are *reinforcing your sickness.* And if you see yourself as sick, as less than whole, then you are energetically accepting their view of you, which makes it that much harder to heal. So, we need to ask that those praying for us see us as whole and healthy, not sick. This reframing addresses the issue from a state of reality about our true being instead of reinforcing a state of illusion.

I only told close family members and a few friends, since I had enough on my plate managing everything that was coming up in me—from the emotions to the change in diet and lifestyle to the fatigue and nausea from treatment. I felt that I didn't want a group of people feeling pity for me because I was dealing with this issue, but again, our situations aren't black and white. We need to accept help, and prayer is at the top of the list. It is also interesting to make note of what I discussed in the preface about how cancer is labeled and viewed. Do we feel a need to tell more people of our diagnosis than if we had depression? Do we tell people what stage we're in, or are we just telling them in general that we have the dreaded "cancer"?

There is a fine line between seeing the world through eyes of separation and what comes with it—sickness, greed, and everyone's being out for themselves—and seeing everything in a state of unity by perceiving someone as whole and complete but with a temporary health issue. This understanding and remembrance is actually a big part of what we're here on Earth to work out. We have to hold a paradox—that everything is whole and complete even if appearances don't reflect that. This unity consciousness is important as it relates to how we view the cancer that is in our body. Do we hate it? Are we angry at it? It will not serve us to see it as separate. It is a part of us, just as our "healthy" cells are a part of us, and we have to come to peace with that—while we work on a treatment plan.

We are whole, but we have to deal with appearances and the consequences that follow from living in a toxic world where our bodies become sick and need "repair." One analogy which could help is to think of your car. When it's new, it needs little maintenance, but when it reaches 30 thousand miles and then especially 60 thousand miles, it begins to need a lot more. If we've used our car in an abusive manner by not giving it regular maintenance, driving it in a rough fashion, or driving it in a harsh environment, it will need repairs much earlier—similar to a body that's been abused with substances or a bad diet. Even if we have taken good care of the car, when it reaches a higher mileage, it will need significant repairs, like the replacement of a transmission. This analogy is similar to when our bodies advance into old age. There is no shame in your car needing repair. Why should there be shame in your body needing repair?

We view our cars differently from our bodies because many judge themselves—based on societal conditioning—when their bodies break down. But there is no difference. The car analogy reflects the world and reality we have to live in, but it doesn't reflect or take away from our wholeness. Unfortunately, many of us have a hard time grasping this concept because we see ourselves in a state of separation as bodies. And we glorify the body and try to keep it young with all kinds of cosmetic enhancements, plastic surgery, and gimmick treatments—like giving your car a supercharged fuel to make it go much faster but with long-term consequences on the engine. We don't properly understand our relationships to our bodies, and this disconnect comes from a much-too-weighted reliance on the mind. Most people see the body as separate but also something that is essential to their identity, so when they are young and beautiful and strong, they feel good about themselves, but as they age, their self-perception changes.

Unless someone examines this false identity, they will become depressed and especially have a hard time when they develop a serious illness and realize their body is decaying. But this inflection point is actually when large changes can happen. When we finally realize our identity outside of our body—whether we call that Spirit or an individual soul—we see something that continues on after the death of the body. The body is an amazing vehicle and truly a temple, but it's not all we are.

My wife, several of my children, and a few close friends have asked me if I feel less than because now, I only have one testicle. (My wife even started calling me "Uniball.") But I don't feel this way because I don't identify with my body as my greater self. I realize this would still hold true if I had no testicles or even a penis, because my manhood is not defined by my body parts. There is so much debate and dissension over the gender-neutral issue, but it is badly misunderstood. We don't have to cut off our body parts to be gender neutral. We only have to balance the masculine and the feminine inside of us and see others in the same way. This is another reason we are here, and it is important to recognize—whether you believe that God created you or you see yourself as a soul that chooses what it will experience on Earth—that there was a choice made at a much higher level of consciousness and awareness to be in a male or female body— and for a few, an androgynous body—for a definite reason. It is hubris for anyone to say what is right or wrong for another person or group of people.

The universe is working for our highest good at so many levels that we don't understand, and so we really can't and mustn't make hard judgments about anything. Sometimes we are blessed with an opening of the clouds, allowing the sun to shine through and illuminate something for us. For instance, I realized that my anti-cancer diet wasn't going to work unless I truly believed with all of my being that it would work. This is the case for everything. But in order to believe that it would work, I had to go through the diet to release the things that were still present deep within my cells, like my emotions and beliefs and the energetics around them. Only then was I able to fully know that the diet would work.

Our body parts, appearance, and our health status don't define us. *You are not less than whole because you have cancer or a major illness. There is not something wrong with you.* When we state that we are whole, we are not denying the reality that we have a temporary health issue. We are just incorporating this temporary reality into a much larger eternal reality.

If we want to heal, we have to do it from the inside out by starting with our own beliefs and changing them. We will know intuitively who to share with about our health issues—and really any details of our life. We have to resist the need to look outside ourselves for our identity and affirmation of who we are.

FALSE BELIEF

NUMBER EIGHT

> ❝ *I CAN KEEP DOING EVERYTHING*
> *I WAS DOING BEFORE* ❞

T HERE HAS BEEN A TREMENDOUS AMOUNT WRITTEN, PROMOTED, and sold regarding the power of the mind. We are told that we can accomplish superhuman feats like running ultramarathons or holding our breath underwater for many minutes, sleeping only a couple of hours a night, fasting for weeks, or scaling rock faces or climbing the highest mountains without proper gear or support. The mind is capable of pushing us through almost anything, which is highly beneficial for children in horribly abusive family situations, since the mind dissociates in order to survive. But when we are an adult, we can make—and need to make—different choices. Just because we can force a superhuman feat doesn't mean that it's smart to do. In fact, it's highly likely it *isn't* smart and that the middle way is best. It also doesn't mean that other people pushing themselves to the limit, or telling you that you can do similar, have healthy belief systems. We can certainly look around the world at those who are put on pedestals and followed for advice and see that many aren't healthy. These people are often in positions of power or control or pressure themselves to achieve superhuman feats because they need some outside validation of their worth.

Life is meant to be lived in balance. When we push an area of ourselves out of balance, something in another area gives, and this dynamic doesn't have good consequences. So, it's not a good idea, while we're in treatment for a major health issue like cancer, to think we can continue with life the exact same way we did previously. Of course, some treatment situations are much less rigorous than others, but in general, treatment for cancer or any type of major health issue is very taxing. I have heard of some individuals who have continued their rigorous work schedules or exercise routines—one of whom even ran a marathon while in treatment—and this stems from a state of wanting to fight back by resisting—and not fully accepting—the situation. You can say, "I am strong, and this will *not* knock me down or change anything." But the reality is that life has already changed with your diagnosis. Denying reality, even partially, is not wise, and it's another example of how easily we can fool ourselves through our beliefs.

If we look at an animal that is injured or sick in some way, it stays mostly in one spot, since innately it knows that this stillness is what it needs to recover. We must honor the need for much greater rest since this inactivity is what our bodies need to heal. If we push through with our mind and continue how we operated before, we are allowing ourselves to fall out of balance and likely causing additional health issues along the way. Walking is very important to me, and I try to do it every day to get exercise and sun exposure. But there were some days that I felt I just didn't have the energy, so I took a nap—and didn't feel guilty about it. I knew that what I was going through was temporary.

As importantly and as mentioned earlier, cancer or a significant health issue is a major wake-up call to get us to STOP and pay attention—to see how we've gotten there and how we have been fooling ourselves by operating in ways that aren't serving our highest good. If we ignore the signs and we continue working long hours, for example—when it's the stress from working long hours that's likely a major contributor to our health issue—there will probably not be good consequences.

My wife grew up in a house where the women were expected to be cleaning and working throughout the day. They are strong workers and excellent cleaners! This lifestyle was ingrained and conditioned into her, and I could really see this pattern every time her mother visited us, when they would clean and do projects together. My wife was dealing with some health issues before and during my cancer treatment, and she was experiencing a lot of fatigue, but she felt guilty doing something so simple as taking a nap and has had to work hard to clear that conditioning. She has repeatedly asked the question, "Why am I so tired?" This question is a product of trying to utilize the mind to steer around the conditioning. But this mindset doesn't work. We have to confront the false beliefs—in her case that she was lazy and not valuable if she wasn't always working—that created the conditioning and then must release them. And it doesn't usually help us to ask why. The reality was that she was tired and had to deal with that, without judgment or guilt, in a way that was best for her health.

Listen to your body and what it needs, and don't allow any false beliefs and conditioning you hold about being lazy or any other belief to interfere in your healing journey.

FALSE BELIEF

NUMBER NINE

> ## *IT'S WEAK TO BE AFRAID*

L IFE BRINGS US A LOT OF POINTERS THAT ARE INTENDED TO help awaken us to greater realities and perspectives beyond the limited ways in which we see ourselves and the world. Understanding our fears is at the top of the list. We each have many individual fears—not having enough money, losing our job, not living up to our own or other's expectations, not being a success, not finding a partner, or getting sick in a pandemic, to name a few. Our fears are multilayered, and we need to keep peeling back the onion. Many fears we are aware of, but many we are not. For instance, our fear that we may not find a partner could be a larger fear that we are not lovable.

Anger is usually not what it seems; fear is often behind it. Carl Jung, the father of analytical psychology, taught us that projection is a very common phenomenon. Our blaming of others is often our own fear or guilt being projected out. Similarly, our judgment of others is self-judgment being projected out; we judge others because they have qualities that we don't like in ourselves and because they have qualities we wish we had in ourselves. Psychology is a complicated arena in which we're operating in literally every moment of our existence, especially since it relates to our own thoughts, which continuously arise from our beliefs. Our thoughts come from our beliefs, and our beliefs are formed by the conditioning and traumas—however severe or implicit—we've been subjected to from our childhoods, from our adult relationships, from society, and from other sources like intergenerational trauma in our DNA.

Why is psychology important? Because as mentioned earlier, cancer is not random, and our emotions and beliefs have played some part in our getting cancer as well as in our ability to heal from it. And for those of us who receive a cancer diagnosis, and to a certain extent for those who love us, we are traumatized by the diagnosis, especially by the fear that arises and that we need to process for many reasons. Fear of death is the foundational pillar of all other fears. Everything relates back to that central fear and to the corollary fear about what will actually happen when we die, which becomes much greater as we advance into our later years. If we are in some way faith-based, then this fear may already be alleviated to a large extent.

After I finished radiation, I realized that I had suffered PTSD and had disassociated to some extent. Disassociation is a normal reaction to any traumatic situation. It is a built-in mechanism that arises for our survival so that we can endure experiences of trauma. We can see this play out in wars and in other similar situations like severely abusive relationships, especially ones that go on for long periods of time. While a cancer diagnosis cannot be compared to war or severely abusive relationships, the effects and implications of a cancer diagnosis usually unfold over many months and into years, and this is highly traumatic in its own way. From the time I was diagnosed and had surgery to the time I finished treatment, more than four months passed, and I wasn't even really at the end of my journey, since I wasn't getting a follow-up scan for another three months to know the status of the cancer. So, in the back of my mind, I was wondering about the effectiveness of the treatment, not allowing me to fully begin healing emotionally.

My treatment took place every weekday for almost a month. By the end I could tell that even in this short period, something in me had begun to shift that was telling me this might be my routine forever. This thinking was of course not logical, but this is what long-term trauma does to us, and I could see how many who were liberated from the concentration camps were unable to believe that their situation had actually changed, much in the way a bird doesn't leave the cage even when the door is opened. Again, the length of my treatment was relatively on the short end, and if you are having to deal with cancer for years, my heart opens in great empathy and compassion for you. This extended treatment and uncertainty takes a huge toll and is likely to create a severe case of ongoing PTSD, which must and can be continually addressed with the right means.

If we haven't worked on ourselves and our emotional patterns and beliefs to a great extent before we get a cancer diagnosis, it will initially be more difficult to process. But it's critical that we recognize our diagnosis as a vehicle, something the universe is using to make us face our fears. How can we recognize our fears before adverse events happen in our life so that we're at a better starting point to deal with them when they happen? By witnessing our emotions and reactions. If we understand that our anger, blame, and self-judgment are usually a projection and we're willing to look at what's creating these reactions, we can ask the universe, or God, or whatever source comforts us, "What is the belief that I have that is creating this reaction in me?" We will start to see patterns and the conditioning that created these beliefs, and when we shine the light of awareness on what we have tried to keep hidden, it will eventually dissolve—because the false cannot be sustained.

So, it is very important that we examine all the emotions and reactions we have regarding our cancer diagnosis and treatment. This introspection starts and ends with our fear of death. If we're willing to dive into this fear, we can then clear so many other fears we have and really transform our lives in the most wondrous way. As the title of this section states, it is false to believe that it is weak to be afraid. Everyone who has a major health issue will feel some degree of fear, likely to a large extent. Almost everyone who is aging will have some degree of fear, even if minor, about what exactly happens at death. Because of the pandemic and other factors happening in a chaotic world, a large majority of people, even young people, are in fear. So, it's not weak to be afraid, nor is it random that having to process fear is happening to you and to a large percentage of the population. It's also not a punishment or a mistake. How can we view anything as a mistake when it's something that can become manna and a gift for us?

But what will *we* do with this understanding of psychology and fear? Most people will either run from the fear, suppress it, deny it in some way, or stifle it with medicators like drugs and alcohol, workaholism, technology, or many other creative ways that man has devised to avoid being still and addressing what is staring him or her in the face. Can we face the fear, be present with it—not be afraid of it—know that adversity builds strength, and work with the fear to heal ourselves? And in the process, can we heal the world? For as we discussed earlier in the book, there exists only one unified field of energy and what one does affects the rest of the whole—the idea that a butterfly flapping its wings in Indonesia has an impact on everything else. This is truly how the universe works. Your cancer diagnosis is not just about you and is truly part of a greater whole. If somehow, we can carry that understanding, it will help us to deal with everything that comes with the cancer journey.

FALSE BELIEF

NUMBER TEN

> ## *I HAVE CANCER*

W E TOUCHED ON LABELS IN THE PREFACE. LABELS ARE NOT only misleading, but they can also define us in a way that is not beneficial for us to be defined. If someone asks me about another person they've never met and I characterize the person as strange or as someone who doesn't conform to society's norms, or even having an unusual appearance, this portrayal would be interpreted by a hundred people in a hundred different ways according to their unique belief systems. So, everything becomes relative.

What does it mean to label someone as having cancer when everyone has active cancer cells in their body? There can be two individuals with the exact same cancer diagnosis regarding the type of cancer and its stage of development, and because of genetics, not even counting environmental factors or diet, these people can experience two different scenarios. One person's cancer could be growing rapidly while the other person's cancer may have remained stagnant at the same level for many years and only discovered by a fluke. If we were to present this scenario to many different doctors, a majority would recommend treatment, but some might advise to take a wait-and-see approach. Even within the subset that recommends treatment, the treatment recommendations would vary somewhat depending on their training and their belief system, both personal and professional. Again, what I am trying to impress upon you is that life and the way we interpret the world inside and outside of us is all relative; so how the doctor defines you or what treatment path you're told to follow cannot be taken as an absolute. Unfortunately, fear makes us want to look for and cling to absolutes to provide some measure of relief and safety—we want to deal with something known instead of something unknown—but arriving at a place of peace, acceptance, and security won't happen if we never address the underlying fear. And why do we fear the unknown when it is *unknown*?

Soon after I began my diet changes, I would look in the mirror and say that I looked and felt great, which I truly did. But then this voice would pop up saying, "Oh, but they tell you that you have cancer." While this was obviously true at some level, if I had energized that thought—which came from outside conditioning and was only a label—and allowed it to become a strong belief that became my frequent reality instead of the reality of feeling and looking good, then I would have created a harder path for myself and likely a different outcome.

Einstein said that everything in life is vibration. The vibration or frequency we're operating at will bring us more of the same. Thus, we want to be highly cognizant of our thoughts, beliefs, and emotions, since they're playing a big part in creating our reality. When we define someone with a label, we are putting them in a box. The problem that arises is that if the person being placed in a box believes this label and that they're confined within the walls of that box, this belief can then be reinforced in a negative cycle. Simply, if we believe we are sick, then the universe brings us more of that.

If we define ourselves as having a health issue that we're temporarily dealing with, we greatly expand the walls of the box and open up much larger avenues for our healing. I am not playing word games here—how you define yourself and your present situation is critical. I would not and did not say to anyone that I was a cancer patient, and my wife and children and close friends did not define me that way either. I said I was dealing with a temporary health issue.

We have to embrace the paradox, which is very hard for most people as it was for me for a long time. The universe is actually one large paradox. A paradox can be defined as a statement or proposition that seems self-contradictory but that is actually expressing a truth. In the paradox we have to simultaneously hold both sides. The paradox around our cancer is that we want something to be different—we want to be completely healthy AND we see ourselves that way—*while* we also understand that it's likely we don't yet fully recognize this truth and that because of this and the fact that we exist in a human body, we may need to take some physical action to address the cancer. Staying in the paradox keeps us in a state where we recognize the unity behind everything, which empowers us to access a much higher perspective for the decision-making process and to access, too, all possibilities for the highest outcome. We live in a world where we have to use labels, and of course at some level of reality you do have "cancer," but at another level of reality, you are whole and perfect. It's another paradox we have to hold, and it's tangential to the one discussed above. But the main takeaway from this chapter is not to define yourself—and also not to let others define you—with some label that puts you in a box and makes it much harder for you to climb out of it.

FALSE BELIEF

NUMBER ELEVEN

> ## *GOD IS PUNISHING ME*

OR

> ## *GOD HAS ABANDONED ME*

W E HAVE EMPHASIZED THE REALITY THAT IN THIS WORLD of shadows, appearances, and labels, there are no absolutes, and everything is relative. If I were to ask one hundred people their definition of God, I would get one hundred different answers. As with everything else in life, we see God through the lens of our own belief system. For instance, if we had an unemotional father who punished us harshly, we will likely see God that same way. Our childhood conditioning plays a large part in how we see God, but then lumped on top of that is societal and religious conditioning. In the Western world, the Judeo-Christian tradition tells us that we have sinned in some way and that we have to atone for this sin in order to redeem favor with God. But this is not what Jesus told us. He told us that God is Love, not the judgmental and vengeful God represented in the Old Testament. Is it not possible that collectively we are evolving spiritually and that Jesus came to reveal a deeper understanding of who God really is?

Unfortunately, because of conditioning, God's love is viewed through a human lens in the contexts of our relationships to our parents and our partners. With our parents, some of them did amazing jobs, while many did not, but in almost all instances, their love was at least a little conditional. In many cases, it was extremely conditional.

God's love is not conditional. There is nothing we can say, do, or think that would stop our Creator from loving us—this is the very definition of "unconditional." It is important to understand that the Bible and inspired texts from other religions have many great seeds of truth which can point us to God, but we cannot and must not take every word literally. For instance, there are some excellent books that have come out in the last 20-30 years by scholars and professors of religion which have shown unequivocally that in the early days of Christianity, there were numerous competing sects all trying to ensure that their message would be the one to continue on. This power dynamic to control the message is evidenced through the letters of some of the early Church fathers who were conservative and wanted to stamp out any "heresy" as well as to establish power through the apostolic line of the church. Some religious scholars believe that many of these writings—including the canonical gospels—were earlier types of literature reminiscent of today's blogs or promotional pieces intended to attract followers and often written as a response to refute another gospel that was circulating.

We don't know the authors of the canonical gospels or when they were written, but we do know from the discovery of the Dead Sea Scrolls and the Nag Hammadi Library that there was a tremendous number of other writings about the life of Jesus and his sayings which were prominent during the first few centuries after his death, some likely written before the canonical gospels. These "apocryphal" gospels were not included in the Bible because the orthodox version of Christianity won out at the council of Nicaea in 325 AD, when the Church elders decided which writings would be included in the official version of the Christian Bible.

The orthodox version of Christianity says that Jesus is the only son of God and that through his death, the sins of the human race would be absolved for those who believed in him. But this message is not what Jesus said in his own words in the four gospels—and especially if one looks at the noncanonical writings produced after his death. Jesus told us we are all sons of God, that we should worship the Father, not him, and that we would *do greater things than him.* That last statement is pretty powerful and has to make one think and question a lot of entrenched narratives.

When Jesus said that no one comes to the Father except through him, he was talking as the Christ, not from his humanity. Jesus was telling us that we need to recognize the Christ in us to come into a full awareness of our divinity and oneness with God. Christ is the one son of God, and each of us is part of that sonship.

Jesus also said that the Kingdom of God is within, which is another extremely powerful statement that points us to our divinity. We are taught by society—or rather, conditioned—not to look within. Our rampant consumerism tells us we need to use all kinds of products and services so that we can find happiness, which is completely false because doing so requires us to look outside ourselves. Only by looking within can we find the joy and answers we are looking for. This understanding is highly relevant to our spiritual journey and our connection with God, and it is highly relevant to everything else in life, especially when we need answers on something as difficult as what steps to take on our cancer journey. As you, the reader, have seen and as I will continue to emphasize, I don't have *your* answers. And no one else does either.

But as we discussed earlier, there are many reasons we don't want to look within. We want to give our power away by abdicating our personal authority and having someone tell us what to do. This abdication is highly applicable to our spiritual journey, since it relates to who we are and what we should believe about God and since, unfortunately, many have given their power to religious or spiritual authorities or gurus. In Christianity, this was not by accident—the church wanted to establish a hierarchy and structure of control and power. If someone knew, as Jesus taught, that you can go directly to God without going through an intermediary, neither the church nor any other religious power structure would exist. There are consequentially many individuals who have become soured at what they were taught about a distant, unreachable, and punishing God in religious schools or other settings, which has unfortunately precluded them from knowing the true God and asking for help.

God is not a punishing God. God is Love. God did not create your cancer, since individually and collectively we have free will. As discussed, with our individual choices it's highly likely we hold at least partial responsibility for being in the situation we are in. Collectively, we have chosen a path of allowing large toxicity to be put in our food, air, and water—literally all of the spaces we inhabit. Even if we have a strong relationship with God, we haven't done something wrong when we get cancer or encounter other adversity in life. I initially questioned, but soon dropped ruminating on, how I could get cancer. Some things just happen in this earth reality that are integrated into our lives as adverse circumstances, regardless of our spiritual connection or how good a life we think we have lived. In these instances, we have to be open to healing our adverse circumstances through all means, including treatments we might have shunned because they were "of the world" and part of the standard Western medical model. We can't just ignore the issue or say we're above it because of our spiritual connection or our faith. Some actually do this, but the consequences are not usually good. The world that man has created can be a very harsh and difficult place—as opposed to what God created and which is so beautiful. But free will means that God doesn't interfere in our affairs.

God did not create your cancer, nor can God cure your cancer— not in the way that most people think of God. God is not separate from you and is not some omnipotent ruler making decisions to bestow or withhold cures or miracles for certain individuals. God is one unified field of energy, as mystics throughout the ages have told us. So, God is expressing through each of us—you, me, Jesus—and all creation. The only difference is our awareness of this. I have been blessed to see God expressing through all creation, but I will admit that as I was on the table in a sterile and cold room with the radiation equipment right over me doing its thing literally a few inches from me, I was challenged to see God in that equipment!

When we say that God is One, this means not only that there is only one God but also that God is all that exists. In this unique reality where we take on a human form, each of us serves as God's hands and feet, and if we want to be healed, we have to take responsibility for our part. God is working in and through us, not separate from us, and we need to acknowledge and affirm this holy reality for the highest healing. God has not abandoned you. This is literally not possible. God is also working through an immense number of helpers, both human and angelic, to encourage us down the right path. Unfortunately, many ignore the signals and pay the consequences.

Because God is holy and perfect and because we are in a state of unity with God, we are holy and perfect. And most of you reading this will immediately think that this is not possible, as you look around at all of the people who are *obviously* not perfect. But I ask that you, for just a moment, remember that you are seeing the world through your own lens and shift your thinking to be completely outside the box.

We live in a world of duality and contrast where everything appears to have an opposite—good and bad, light and dark, black and white. But there is really nothing that is black and white. Everything is relative and flows on one continuum, blending to gray—this is the reason that labels are so misleading. Through our discussions earlier about what science has shown us about the nature of the universe, we can see that there is no separation. Everything is relational and in a state of constantly changing energy.

The Kingdom of God is based on unity. There are no degrees—only the appearance of degrees. If I ask one hundred people their definition of sin, I will get 100 different answers, because there is no standard accepted definition—the definition of sin and our perception about all existence is relative, not absolute. But something absolute—God, that is—must be behind all appearances. So, back to my statement that you are holy and perfect. What is the level of perfection that we can reach? How kind or smart do we have to become? But can't we become even kinder after we reach that destination? Wouldn't some people still say we weren't kind? Whose opinion is *true*? Was Jesus imperfect because he harbored anger, grief, and doubts? Would we ever say that a painting or the way a bird sings is imperfect?

We wouldn't, and the same holds true for us. Perfection is simply the expression of God through us and all creation. It is not a destination. Nor is our holiness up for debate, even if you think you have "sinned" and thus violated your holiness. We have all certainly made many mistakes, but again, can it be called a mistake if it teaches us how to do it differently the next time? Everything is nuanced, and the paradox is where we hold two seemingly incongruent positions. We have the attributes of God, but in this earth reality where the appearance of separation creates duality, we must "improve" and make amends, forgive, and "better" ourselves. We are already at a destination, but we're also working towards a destination. What I mentioned in the last section—accepting ourselves as whole *while* working to heal ourselves—gives us the greatest chance at success.

Of course, there are large numbers of people committing heinous acts that come from an ignorance of their divinity or from an active rebellion against God. They are also a part of God, but this truth does not excuse their actions, and we must deal with their actions appropriately. Jesus said to give to Caesar the things that are Caesar's and to give to God the things that are God's, which means that we have to deal with the world we live in. As we accept the world we live in while at the same time desiring positive change and working towards it—what we need to do with our health issues—we hold the paradox and the higher understanding that will help us to see our "problems," such as a cancer diagnosis, in a completely different light. This enlarged perspective places us in a powerful concurrent state of acceptance, surrender, and knowledge of right action for our healing. It enables us to bring in many additional spiritual and emotional tools for healing, as well as to be open to and to be able to feel at a much deeper level what physical tools like treatments and therapies we need.

How can we enter into communion with God where we can access that help? One of the impediments to knowing God is that we are heavily mind-centered in Western society. This imbalance has been worsened by religious scholars who analyze each word of scripture from every angle, issuing theological dissertations on what a given passage means, making assumptions about Jesus' life—all through their logical minds—to an unquestioning acceptance by many people. We can only *think* God through our minds. What we want is to *experience God.* In order to know God at the level of Spirit and to have an experience of that love and communion which is outside of the mind, we have to use our hearts. We have to listen to that still small voice. When some people think they hear God, they are actually using their logical minds. Few people are willing to put down the technology and be still long enough to hear God, who is talking to us *all of the time.* There is no end to our deepening into God, who is infinite and eternal. So if we think we have all the answers, we don't; we're engaging in spiritual hubris. Socrates said "The only true wisdom is in knowing you know nothing."

Jesus said that the meek shall inherit the earth and that one must be like a little child to enter the Kingdom. Think of the innocence, non-judgment, pure joy and trust that little children carry. They're not analyzing everything. They're not trying to achieve anything or worried about how others see them. They are just in the moment doing their thing—until they are conditioned by society and well-meaning but misguided parents. Little children can show us the way, teaching us about the spiritual journeys that are so integral to our cancer or health journeys. No one can take our cancer journey or our spiritual journey for us. We have to show up and face it head on using all the tools at our disposal that God has given us. With our health journeys and everything we face in life, we can't use a wrench when we need a screwdriver, which is what we do when we want to get out of fear as quickly as possible and use only our minds to make decisions.

If you are not asking God for help in dealing with your health issue—from physical, emotional, mental, or spiritual healing to patience to faith—you are missing out on a huge opportunity to ease your path, to open the door for miracles and blessings, and to come to know God's love and comfort at a deep level.

I continually stress our belief systems, even using false beliefs as the chapter title, because it can be so beneficial. But the flipside is that it can be detrimental to our healing. This is why I have spent most of this chapter discussing the importance of our spiritual foundation. I strongly suggest that you ask yourself what it is that you truly believe about God. Where did those beliefs come from? What type of conditioning did you experience that created this belief in you?

If you don't believe in the existence of God or a Creator, why not? The answer that many normally give is that there is no proof of God. But I would say to show me the proof that God *doesn't* exist. If I asked one hundred people—yes, I know I'm continually returning to this "ask one hundred people" track!— who call themselves atheists, keeping in mind that, again, labels are misleading, what it would take to prove to them that God exists, I would get one hundred different answers. It's all relative and always changing. Actually, many would not be able to give an answer. Or maybe they'd only believe God exists if an old white male with a beard and crown, sitting on a throne throwing thunderbolts or performing miracles—again, conditioning from religion—appeared before them. But if this actually happened, many of those witnessing it would make excuses seeking to explain why this wasn't valid—temporary hallucination or a projected hologram from someone trying to fool them, for example. For when we are resistant to changing our beliefs, there is no amount of evidence that will be satisfactory. This truth is extremely evident in the world we live in and in the ways people are split to one side or the other, especially in the last few years. St. Thomas Aquinas, an influential Dominican friar and priest as well as a theologian and philosopher in the Middle Ages, said it best: "To one who has faith, no explanation is necessary. To one without faith, no explanation is possible."

FALSE BELIEF

NUMBER TWELVE

> *I CAN HEAL THIS ON MY OWN WITHOUT CONVENTIONAL TREATMENT*

T HIS FALSE BELIEF IS NOT INTENDED TO BE A COMPLETELY encompassing statement, as there are certainly cases where people have healed even late-stage cancers without conventional treatment—and the flipside where others have healed late-stage cancers with only conventional treatment. Unfortunately, we are often told about these people by others who have a vested interest in seeing us go down the same path, usually for monetary purposes. Perhaps they want to sell us their experience and belief system in some way. This doesn't mean that these people who have monetized their or other's experiences didn't start out with good intentions or that they don't still have them, but they believe what they believe, right? Again, our beliefs and other's beliefs are foundational for us to examine. And money and reputation can have a way of taking someone down a path where they justify what they promote without being willing to incorporate other paths, like diet or treatment modalities, for example. This absolutism is no different for those who promote conventional treatment as the only way.

In order to heal pronounced, active-tumor cancer without conventional treatment, we have to be of a certain mindset and makeup. Unfortunately, not that many are of this mindset, and few are good at evaluating whether they are of this mindset. Thus, they listen to what others say and give their power away. We can listen to others without giving our power away, and to a certain extent it is likely that we do want to listen to others' opinions, especially considering treatment options in different areas ranging from the conventional to the alternative. But we need to do this without automatically accepting something because it comes from a certain source or because it aligns with what we have always believed. The process of gathering information, sorting through the emotions that arise, and having patience is critical in order to make the decision that is right for us. If this process still includes the path of healing without conventional treatment, it is important to recognize our thought process. Our mind will affirm that we can achieve this, and it's likely that we are excited about the prospect of treating naturally, which is not in and of itself a "bad" thing. But most people aren't able to heal their cancer themselves, and then when it spreads, they become very fearful and rush into conventional treatment. If they had started conventional treatment earlier, they might have been able to jump on top of it and might have had a much better prognosis. Panic is never a good state to be in when trying to heal.

It is important to remember that we are all highly unique in our genetics, lifestyles, environmental exposures, toxic loads, and especially our mental, emotional, and spiritual mindsets. So, when someone says they have healed cancer on their own using this or that diet, supplement, program, or therapy, it's not comparable to anyone else's situation. And even if we're told in specifics what this person did daily, it's still incomplete information. Are we told whether they had a very supportive spouse? Are we told if they work in a family business and were able to cut back their hours significantly? This doesn't in any way mean that the information others give us about their treatment journey isn't valuable. It's just important to understand that at best, it's only partially applicable to someone else.

The biggest takeaway I want to stress is that you can only be successful in healing cancer on your own if *you believe you can with every fiber of your being.* This is the power of the mind and our beliefs. For we will fool ourselves into thinking that we can heal cancer without conventional treatment and we will think that we *can* make ourselves believe we are capable of believing this with every cell in our body when that's usually not the case. As we mentioned earlier, knowing thyself is one of the keys to life and our growth here. If we know ourselves to a great extent, we won't be able to fool ourselves. For the reality is that a large majority of people will have some doubt about whether they can accomplish healing without conventional treatment. *This is human nature.* It's not something to feel ashamed or guilty about if we determine we can't do this, although for many that doubt is not likely present in their consciousness where they can recognize it. If we can recognize this, we can feel grateful we have this awareness. But there is a small subset of people who have an innate knowing that anything is possible, and they live life this way. They can serve as a great example for the rest of us. They are able to live without the fear that what they're doing isn't working. And so, they're able to heal cancer without conventional treatment, although it will usually take an extended period— which in some way they have come to terms with as well.

One of the reasons I waited on deciding a course of treatment is that I wasn't sure about whether I could heal my cancer on my own. While many people will panic and jump right into conventional treatment to try and alleviate the fear, I was blessed in that I had already worked on healing fear enough in my life to recognize it and not let it overtake me or especially my decision-making process. When we can recognize we are in fear, we need to stop and refrain from making any decisions until we're out of fear. In addition, I knew that if I just asked God, the answer would be provided to me, because I've been fortunate to learn patience with my spiritual growth. In fact, with the diagnosis after surgery that cancer was still there, I had to use many of my tools that I had accumulated over the years—not falling into fear, trust, listening to my body, not allowing others' energetics and wishes to influence me, and patience—allowing the answer to flow into me in a gentle way, which is how the universe works.

I wasn't looking for a specific answer, since I had also learned that sometimes the answer is something I least expect or is an answer that didn't occur to me as a possible path. These answers can be the best kind because they truly come from a deeper place of wisdom. The obvious two answers in this case for most people would be whether they get conventional treatment or not, and if so, when the best time to start would be. This decision was somewhat the case for me, but it was more expansive, since I was looking for an answer as to whether I could *know* with every fiber of my being that I could heal my cancer on my own. I define knowing in this case as a much deeper level of wisdom than believing, because our beliefs change almost every moment as new input comes in. They change if we are open to change itself, which is a fluid state of being and how we are intended to walk the world. So I needed to see whether I could align all of my body, mind, and spirit—every part, every cell, and all of my consciousness into healing my cancer. And I determined that I could not.

We are meant to be in the world but not of it, and it's not only possible that we can heal things within ourselves; this possibility can become a reality, just as an acorn has the DNA to become a massive oak tree. But when reality meets expectations or super lofty goals, we have to make a proper analysis of where we're at. Even with my long history of emotional and spiritual healing and growth and with my close relationship with God, I determined that healing cancer without conventional treatment was not possible for me at this time. I knew there would be some lingering doubt that would prevent this from happening, potentially putting me in a worse situation. I don't think I was fearful in any way, since I had surrendered to whatever outcome. I just think this path was the one that presented itself—and who knows, maybe one of the reasons was because I was meant to write this book to help others.

Ideally, we would live in a world where the best of conventional and alternative treatments, diet, faith, and mind-body and other holistic practices would be integrated and would provide the patient a true path for healing using all tools. But we don't live in this type of world. This world is one of polarities and extremes, evidenced by so many other issues outside of health. Unfortunately, we can't expect our oncologist to talk to us about diet or acupuncture or faith or wireless technology. But this should collectively be our goal as we continue to always work towards balance and a higher perspective.

As we repeatedly discuss in the book, look at your beliefs and begin to know thyself. Get quiet and still so you can deal with the feelings and give yourself the space and time to make a decision that is in your highest good. If it is in your highest good, it will be in the highest good for those you love and actually, too, for the whole world, because only one highest good exists. That highest good is one of joy, peace, and love. You may have some obstacles to overcome to get there, but these obstacles build the inner strength that accompanies the joy, peace, and love.

FALSE BELIEF

NUMBER THIRTEEN

> *I CAN'T BE GRATEFUL OR JOYFUL WHEN ADVERSE THINGS HAPPEN TO ME*

G RATITUDE IS A PART OF OUR DIVINE INHERITANCE AND A natural attribute of our unity with God, but in this world of duality, where there is contrast between "good" and "bad" choices and states of being, at times we have to will ourselves to be grateful. It is easy to fall into self-pity and victimhood with the conditioning that we've received from various sources. Unfortunately, victimhood is celebrated and has become entrenched as acceptable in our society. We can see this reality show up in the billboards telling us we're victims and should be compensated for being wronged or injured, the reinforced delineation of individuals and groups into oppressors and victims, and how we play the victim role as a control mechanism in our personal relationships. When we project out our guilt and self-judgment, we're looking for someone to blame. While in many instances assigning responsibility is important, there is a fine line between holding others accountable and falling into victimhood. Our actions and words always need to come from compassion and a willingness to discuss things in a way that can be resolved for the highest good of everyone. As a society discussing numerous sensitive issues, this means we don't switch oppressor and victim roles, since that back-and-forth keeps us in the same destructive cycle. Obviously, operating from a perspective above oppressors and victims is far from the state of our world today.

Gratitude is a mental and especially an emotional and spiritual muscle we have to exercise, much like going to the gym to work on our physical bodies. Because we live in a difficult world and we encounter many adverse situations related to ourselves and those we love, almost everyone falls into self-pity at times. But we can't stay there, since doing so creates a pattern that turns into victimhood. We have discussed energetics throughout the book. Self-pity, resentment, and victimhood are contracting states, while gratitude is an expansive state. If we're in resentment about our cancer diagnosis or the treatment we have to undertake, we're not in a good place to be for healing. We need expansive states of gratitude, optimism—balanced with reality—joy, and love in order to heal. For when we are in states of expansion, we more closely align with the wholeness and resonance of unity and God, which is perfect health. Again, the paradox is that we're not there, since we're still dealing with a health issue. But we have to simultaneously hold the paradox of where we are and who we know ourselves to be.

The reality of being on Earth in a human body is that you'll have "adverse" things happen to you, just as you'll have "amazing" things happen to you—like getting a big raise or a new love relationship. "Adverse" and "amazing" are in quotation marks because these labels are relative and dependent on our judgment system. Many experiences that are initially deemed as adverse are looked at later as gifts that we're grateful for when we realize that we were forced into a change that we had been resisting but that was good for us. This also usually entails a new awareness about ourselves, others, the world, and the nature of God, to name a few. Having flexibility in our belief system broadens our perspective, allowing us to soften our judgments and to see that nothing is completely black and white. It allows us to see more from a unitive perspective than from a separatist one.

What we don't want to do is be so hardened in our beliefs that we fail to grow and that life tosses us around like a rag doll that is in a dog's mouth. If we stay in a state where we see only separation and don't recognize the unity that is behind all appearances, we're being tossed around on the waves of the ocean of life. Life is battering us, and we don't have a boat or a life preserver. If we see from a higher perspective, then we balance the ups and downs. We don't get depressed or angry when our sports team loses or when we don't get the promotion. We are grateful, not excited in an ego-based way, when something amazing happens for us. Ego excitement is based on circumstances of the world going well for us, although this false joy is always temporary and will be replaced by something that depresses us—because we are chasing and looking to what is false to be our god. We are chasing some type of destination we probably can't even elucidate and one that would likely not satisfy us even if we achieved it, like having some particular amount of money or being at a certain level in our career.

When we operate with an understanding of the divine flow and the gifts that are our inheritance, there is an undercurrent of joy behind the gratitude. This joy comes from God and never goes away. It is there even when we are undergoing adverse circumstances like cancer treatment. Having this connection with God and operating in gratitude and joy does not mean that we don't temporarily experience fear as well as grief as we process what is happening to us. They are not mutually exclusive. Again, this perspective may sound paradoxical, and it is, but this holding of multiple realities is how we need to operate.

The reality is that being cured of cancer will not give us true joy. It is just another up that would accompany the down—that is, our cancer diagnosis. Granted, they are large ups and downs compared to our sports team winning or losing, but the principle still applies. Our joy is not dependent on *anything*—any event, any experience, any outcome, or *anyone* outside of us.

Connecting with our inherent gratitude and joy allows us to receive much greater awareness for options for our healing. It allows us to be at peace with what we're experiencing and at peace with all potential outcomes.

Gratitude is an energetic state that is felt in the body. The mind will be a witness to when we are in a self-pitying or victim mentality, and if we're in tune with our body, this sensation won't feel good. But we need to quickly move from the mind to the heart and body. I see and especially feel my heart opening like a beautiful flower, and I can feel the expansion within me.

If we find ourselves unable to get into a state of gratitude, we can start by practicing the simplest of recognitions, such as the fact we are alive, that we can read these words, and that we have someone in our life who loves us. We are geared in our DNA and our spiritual body to move quickly to gratitude, so once we start practicing it, the exercise will be like riding a bike. We just have to be consistent in doing it, since we're re-forming neural pathways that may have been dormant for a long time.

With my cancer treatment, I was grateful that I had various treatment options to consider, from conventional treatment to diet and more. Even though my urologist and radiation oncologist viewed my path forward through a fairly narrow lens informed by their conditioning from medical training, I could see that they really cared about people and that they're just human beings doing the best job they can, as we all are. I didn't judge them because they were promoting conventional treatment, which I had previously judged to some degree. It's amazing and such a blessing how the universe gives us opportunities to see how our beliefs come from judgment in ways that don't serve our highest good. Having cancer allowed me to write this book and to move to an even higher perspective in many areas. As mentioned earlier, it brought me to a much greater state of compassion for myself, those in the medical establishment, and those undergoing significant health challenges. The compassion opened my heart so that I could know the best path for myself and could then possibly be of service to others undergoing similar challenges. Even the most adverse set of circumstances can be turned into beauty, holiness, and immense opportunities for growth depending on how we react to those circumstances.

FALSE BELIEF

NUMBER FOURTEEN

> ## *CANCER HAS INTERRUPTED MY LIFE*

B ELIEVING THAT CANCER HAS INTERRUPTED OUR LIFE DEPENDS on how we see the world. Are we a glass-half-empty or glass-half-full person? If we see the cancer diagnosis and the treatment protocol that follows as a pain in the butt, then we'll believe that it has interrupted our life. We are operating in the realm of "good" and "bad," which we previously touched on, and within this belief system, we may stay angry and depressed about our cancer until we're finished with treatment and are cleared, at which point we'll be excited or relieved and want to put it in the past. But when we do this, we're fooling ourselves. The cancer is just appearing as a larger manifestation of a central underlying problem, which is that we see life through "good" and "bad." I use the word "appearing" because the cancer is no different from shingles, a broken foot, or a severe sinus infection—just "worse" in our own mind because these other examples are not likely to kill us. We tend to assign value judgments and degrees thereof, especially when it comes to our health and the potential for an issue to be fatal. But within unity there are no degrees, and this reality aligns with someone who has a glass-half-full perspective in that they are always looking for silver linings in the most adverse circumstances.

If we use cancer as a vehicle for a higher understanding, it completely alters how we view life and dealing with an experience like cancer. We can view our life from a treetop perspective, seeing that the forest consists of many trees—along with birds, other animals, and a mix of greens and browns. Most of us are on the floor of the forest with our faces pressed up against the trunk of a tree, and we think life is only this brown scaly surface we can perceive. With a treetop perspective we can fit our cancer diagnosis and journey into a much larger puzzle, seeing a flow and a purpose to our life that helps us to understand how we got to where we are and where we may be going.

A minority of people—but a growing one!—take the time to ask the big questions in life. These are the ones that have true meaning, not questions like "Where should we go on vacation this year?" or "How can I advance in my career?" It's not that questions like these don't need to be asked; it's just that they're very secondary to much larger questions. When we ask the larger questions, we will *receive the larger answers.* This is one of the reasons we are here on Earth. Asking the larger questions allows our cancer journey to fit within a framework and paradigm that we can understand and accept. This is why I counsel to refrain from making rushed decisions around anything, especially our cancer treatment. It helps to be asking the larger questions from a state of awareness where we can process the answers with both our gut and our conscious mind. If we are not yet there, we are being pushed to get there by many vehicles.

FALSE BELIEF

NUMBER FIFTEEN

> ## I CAN'T DO THIS

T HE VEHICLES THAT SHOW UP IN OUR LIVES—HEALTH challenges, relationships, and experiences, for example— don't have to be "negative" as we define it but we could find ourselves facing adversity if we have resisted signals and hints that the universe has been giving us and we're living in a toxic world where we have to deal with detrimental decisions and paths that the human race and the collective have taken us down, or some combination of the two.

For many good reasons, humans have a large aversion to pain or negative vehicles of any kind, whether physical, emotional, or mental. Our entrepreneurial society has produced countless hacks to work around and avoid states like pain, sadness, fatigue, or mental fogginess, but this shortcutting is not wise, since we're not allowing natural processes to take their course, which can have disastrous long-term consequences. As part of the human condition, pain—physical, emotional, mental, and spiritual— is unavoidable. And like everything, it can serve our growth in many ways or simply alert us that something is wrong and needs addressing in a healthy way. So, we shouldn't try to avoid these "negative" vehicles or try to hack our way around them as our ego minds would prefer to do. A higher part of us has chosen a path for what we want to accomplish on Earth for our growth. If we avoid a vehicle, it'll likely come up repeatedly and often in a stronger way until we've addressed it. For instance, someone may continually enter into relationships with abusive partners, never seeing the pattern that the story is not about the other person but rather about their own self-worth. Or the vehicle may change to show that person they hold a low self-worth. Not paying attention to what the pain is trying to show us means that we will likely have to be shaken even harder the next time. Again, the universe or God is not punishing us but is instead just fulfilling the growth we have asked for at a level far outside our limited ego mind, which looks through a lens of punishment and can't understand why some given adverse event is happening or continues to happen.

The universe has an innate wisdom and is constantly adjusting to where we are and what we need. It's also showing us that we are much stronger than we can envision. Similar to a parent, boss, or professor who pushes us in a good way, the universe will never give us more than we can handle, for the purpose is for us to succeed. Thus, when we're faced with a challenge, we know that we can handle it. It may look like tapping on reserves of strength that we didn't know we had, and it may push us to the point of exhaustion or extreme grief, but if we can trust in a bigger picture, we can handle what we're going through. Cancer can be one vehicle to show us what we're made of, but there are many others, too, like the breakup of a relationship or the loss of our job or our house. And only we can determine whether that vehicle has presented itself because we've disregarded previous signals or whether it's just a part of being in a highly dysfunctional and toxic world. Often, it's a combo of both. But the reality is that the vehicle is there, and it is meant to serve us, if we allow it, regardless of why it is there.

How do we pull from those inner reserves and make it through? By taking one day—literally one moment—at a time. With cancer we have to compartmentalize our schedule and treatment, not looking ahead. So on the day of my surgery, I only thought about a series of the smallest successive steps without jumping to the next one: get in the car with my wife, get checked in, get in the hospital bed, and give my arm for my IV, for example. I wasn't thinking how much pain I would be in after surgery, how the dog would get walked every day, or if the surgery was going to clear the cancer. When I had radiation treatment every weekday for almost a month, it just became routine that I had to get up and go there each morning, just like I brushed my teeth. Being at the facility became a series of small steps that I was familiar with after the first visit.

As briefly touched on, staying in the moment, or the now, is a powerful spiritual practice. The present moment is all that exists. Quantum physics has shown us that time is neither fixed nor linear. Einstein told us that "the distinction between the past, present, and future is only a stubbornly persistent illusion." So when we are worrying about potential outcomes for our health issue, we are living in the future, and this is not where we want to be, because we will be in fear. If we stay in the present moment, we stay where God resides and where we can receive answers. If we witness our thoughts and watch how they drift to the future regarding what will happen to us—our loved ones, the world, or anything else—we can bring them back to the present moment and remind ourselves to be here, right now, in this body. Being in the present moment allows us to compartmentalize all of these moments into one after the other so we're not being overwhelmed by fear of the future.

One of my strengths is logic, which I have learned to balance with the heart. Logic tells us that we can do something because we have to do it, since we don't have another choice. We actually do have other choices than to face what is in front of us, but denial is never a good path and usually leads to far worse outcomes than if we had just had the courage to face the issue to begin with.

Yes, cancer has in some way interrupted our life, but as we discussed earlier, this is *a good thing*, and if we so choose, we can see it this way, recognizing the gifts and needed changes it brings. Many choose not to and don't process the emotions, just wanting to get through it as quickly as possible. If we are grateful for the gifts that bring a higher perspective and if we combine this gratitude with logic that tells us that we are here—so we must deal with our adversity because it's not going away—we are invited to surrender to the fact that we are not in control of things as we thought we were. This relinquishment of control brings us to a beautiful place of inner peace. When we let go of control, magic happens.

When I was diagnosed with cancer, I would have obviously preferred not to have it. But I didn't panic, and I surrendered to the fact I needed surgery, which is all I could know at that point. I went through the surgery keeping my focus on what the next thing right in front of me was that I needed to do or not do. I didn't worry about whether the surgery would be the end of my cancer journey—whether it had spread to other areas—since there was zero benefit in worrying at all, especially worrying about something I could not control and would not have information about until later.

We need to control the things we can control and give what we can't control to God. The issue lies in determining what we can control. It is highly likely that we think we can control much more than we really can. Because we are not good judges of what we can and cannot control, the safest route is to assume we can't control anything—which knocks down the ego and creates humility—and to give it all to God. We can desire that we would not want to experience the cancer journey *while* understanding that we are not in control, which then allows us to accept and not resist what we desire we do not have—the principal paradox.

Of course, at a level of Spirit, we work hand in hand with God to fulfill our soul's choices, so that is the ultimate control. But not many people walk the earth from the same consciousness and recognition of unity that Jesus did. So, it is best to assume that we don't know what is in our best interest and that we can't control anything. Nor should we compare ourselves to others—I could have easily become angry that I got cancer when my diet and lifestyle choices were vastly healthier than those of a large percentage of the population. We can't figure it out, so we must give it all to God. With that surrender comes great peace and joy. The Serenity Prayer says it best: "God, grant me the serenity to accept the things I cannot change, courage to change the things I can, and the wisdom to know the difference, living one day at a time; enjoying one moment at a time; taking this world as it is and not as I would have it..."

I quickly accepted that I needed some changes in my life regarding diet, the use of technology, and more. Although these changes were substantial, especially with the diet and the juicing, I didn't panic. Because I was in the moment, I was able to feel how I needed to stage out changes without them becoming overwhelming, and there were many things that I realized that I just couldn't do, since they would have been too much on my plate. Self-analysis of what we can handle and what our body needs, but without fear, guilt, or self-judgment, is critical. But we all need time, patience, and compassion to be able to make this self-analysis.

When I had a CT scan after my surgery and the enlarged lymph node showed up, I was temporarily rocked. But then I knew that staying in any state of self-pity or denial would not be beneficial. I also knew that I have tremendous inner strength I could call on, buttressed by immense faith and trust. So, I quickly accepted that this was my new normal for at least a certain time—I had my "regular" normal before surgery, a new normal with the month-long recovery from the surgery, and now this, which would be an even newer normal. Again, as humans we want to label things and put them in boxes so we can process— theoretically—and deal with them more easily, but the universe has a good laugh at our need to segment and control our lives, since change is the only constant.

Then when I started radiation and had to be at the treatment center every weekday for almost a month, I just accepted what was and didn't look ahead or back. By the time I was nearing the end of the treatment, I was so exhausted that I was counting down the last segment in days, but I was able to be in the moment from the time I was driving over, to sitting in the lobby, to undressing and putting on my gown, to the 35 to 45 minutes I was on the table as I received the radiation in four areas. I joked with my main radiation tech that I had come there for the ambiance, which comprised the flashing lights, the laser, and the rock music they played at my request. I didn't want to be there, but I also didn't resist it in any part of my being. Here we see the paradox again. I made the best of it by really appreciating and thanking those who were treating me and by being grateful that my insurance covered most of this treatment, among other perspectives. The little things and staying in the moment helped me to see God in all things, including everything around this journey, and to tap into my inner strength to get through what was a traumatic experience.

If someone is looking ahead to the day they're cancer-free—and, again, what does this even mean?—they are not living life. They are waiting for something in the future they think will be a better situation for them, similar to the way someone who is constantly moving to new jobs or relationships keeps thinking that the grass is greener on the other side. In some ways it may be, but in other ways it wouldn't, because the richness and joy of life is in the moment, not in looking ahead to a time when we believe we will be happier. And what if that time of being cancer-free never comes?

If you have cancer or some major health issue, or if a loved one has it, what good is it to be non-accepting of the situation? Yes, we have to go through the stages of grief I previously outlined, but after that, we need to stay in a place of surrender. Being in any other state won't change the reality of the situation or help us to heal. Surrender means accepting that you may be dealing with cancer for the rest of your life or the possibility that your physical body may not make it, but that your spirit will go on. You can't live fully unless you're not afraid of dying.

Surrender is the thread that needs to be present in and for all of our cancer and other health journeys and especially throughout our lives. There are numerous testimonials of individuals who healed themselves of late-stage cancers using a plant-based or other type of alternative diet. But many of these individuals had been through conventional treatment without success, and they turned to a specific diet and other therapies in desperation or as a last resort. What actually happened is that they surrendered, and out of that surrender came a cure... because they allowed for all possibilities. The diet was important, but it was their change of attitude and the releasing of false beliefs and blocks, the releasing of the belief that they were in control, that then allowed the diet and other treatments to work to the highest degree. There is a high potential for miracles to happen for each of us if we are open to it.

FALSE BELIEF

NUMBER SIXTEEN

> *EVERYONE SHOULD DO CHEMOTHERAPY*

O NCOLOGY DRUG REVENUE REACHED $176 BILLION IN 2021, more than double the next class of drugs. This is big business. But just because something is being widely used, it doesn't mean that it's necessarily the best option for everyone, especially when money is involved. As we've already discussed, we live in a corporatocracy.

I'm not here to tell you what to do. As has become evident throughout the book, I am pointing you back inside yourself to determine what is best for you. I can only share my experiences in the hope that they are beneficial to you. Certainly, where I have experienced something, as is the case with most of what I have written over the years, there is greater credibility to it. For instance, I have experienced and healed a great deal of fear that had its origin in sexual abuse by my mother, so I feel like I am in a much better position to talk about it—and write a book on it—than someone who just learns about it in school. There is a world of difference between experience and what is generated solely by the mind, and this truth gets continually reinforced to me in experiences like my cancer diagnosis and treatment, for example. When we experience it, we are now truly walking in someone else's shoes and doing so generates a lot of compassion for us and for them. I stay quiet about things I have not experienced, such as homelessness or having to live paycheck to paycheck.

So, when I speak of chemotherapy, I have not experienced it directly, although I have seen and been around others who have gone through treatment. With my radiation treatment there were chemo patients also undergoing radiation in the same facility. I am extremely blessed that up to this point, even though my urologist was recommending I do it, I have not had to consider chemotherapy, since my cancer wasn't late stage.

Studies through the National Institutes of Health (NIH) have shown that those undergoing certain types of radiation and chemotherapy treatment have a higher likelihood of having future secondary cancers that are not necessarily related to the first cancer that was treated, so there is a trade-off between living now, living well, living without fear, and living later. For each person this will be unique and *only you can make this decision for yourself.* But we should not make any decision hastily. Rare is the person who can immediately feel from the deepest part of their being and know the best path to take. For the vast majority, a quick decision is almost certainly being made from a space of fear and the desire to get a solution as quickly as possible.

There are obviously certain types of cancers that are well-suited to radiation, like a cancer that's contained in one organ or lymph node. If cancer has metastasized, I understand the logic behind needing to suppress it through chemotherapy that is systemwide, but I don't know that the tradeoffs and risks are being properly evaluated. I believe that in most cases, a chemo oncologist is just telling patients, "You need to do this, and these will be your potential side effects."

For the sake of an example, If I have a lawn full of weeds and there are too many to pull up manually, I can spray them with a poison to kill the weeds (though we haven't sprayed our yard in many years). But this poison is going to kill the healthy grass that's near the weed and sprayed at the same time. Systemic chemotherapy seems to me to be far worse, as it is spraying the poison over the whole body—analogous to the lawn—not just selectively, with the hope that all of the cancer cells, the weeds, die and enough healthy cells, or the grass, can survive. The scenario in which all weeds are killed and the lawn is able to regenerate itself in a completely healthy way seems logically unlikely to me. A more likely scenario is that many of the weeds die, but some mutate or go dormant, and we have negatively altered the microbiome—the microorganisms in a particular environment—of the whole lawn, possibly forever. I'll add here that the lawn example is not ideal, since weeds in a lawn are actually indicative of what is naturally occurring and healthy, but I think you can understand how I'm using this example.

A much better approach seems to be that we aid the microbiome of the lawn by introducing treatments that will naturally inhibit growth of the weeds and promote growth of the grass. We can see similarities for the treatment of our body through many of the ways we have already discussed—like diet, supplements, addressing our lifestyle, and environmental factors, for example.

I am not telling anyone not to get chemotherapy. My heart goes out to those who are faced with a difficult decision if they have late-stage cancer and need to knock it back. What I am saying is that there are many factors here that need to be considered, especially if you do not have late-stage cancer but rather one that would be treated effectively by radiation, which can be more targeted. There are also, obviously, many who have late-stage cancer who have opted not to undergo chemotherapy and its side effects so that they have some quality of life in their remaining time. Again, we need not to make a rushed decision, especially one to jump into treatment quickly due to our fear. After we have done all the research and had all of the conversations with various doctors and health experts, friends, and loved ones, we need to sit with not only all of the info and all of the possibilities for treatment paths, but also with all of the possibilities when God is involved. It is then we can feel what is best for us, at which point we need to take the path that feels good to our heart and body—and to every part of our being—with the complete certainty that this direction that has been shown to us is the path of our highest good. This will bring peace, for we have done all we can do.

FALSE BELIEF

NUMBER SEVENTEEN

> ## *I WANT TO CURE MY CANCER*

WE DON'T WANT TO CURE OUR CANCER. WE WANT TO heal it. As I am defining it, healing encompasses a much broader perspective. It encompasses everything we have discussed in this book. Healing involves many realms beyond the physical—namely emotional, mental, energetic, and spiritual. Obviously, we would prefer that it does, but healing may or may not include a physical "cure." But it is likely we will have a physical cure if the other areas mentioned above are brought into a state of integration and wholeness, since our energetics greatly impact our physical health. But we need to be prepared for and surrender to whatever the outcome turns out to be. If we have completely surrendered, then tremendous healing beyond the physical has already occurred.

I propose a six-step healing cycle, some of which we have reviewed in parts. This cycle has been highly beneficial for me, and it can be beneficial for anyone processing all of the emotions that have come up around their cancer diagnosis. But it is really applicable in all aspects of our lives. The first step in the cycle is one of inquiry and intention. As if we were a different person, we witness our reactions, thoughts, and feelings, honoring them by not suppressing them, judging them, or cutting them off prematurely. A good starting place is noticing when we have some type of quick emotional reaction or a thought that keeps reoccurring. If we catch it quickly and we witness ourselves having this reaction or thought before it gets into a trail of thoughts—and actually witnessing how one thought leads to another and then to another is a great practice—we can ask why we're having this intense reaction or what the emotion behind this recurring thought is. The emotion that's behind our reaction or behind the recurring thought is usually fear disguised in different ways, maybe as anger or as blame through the vehicle of projection onto others or the world.

The second step in the cycle is to ask to become aware of the false belief that is supporting this reaction or recurring thought, as well as the conditioning that created this false belief, so that we can bring awareness to what is not serving us. Sometimes we know quickly what the false belief is and the conditioning that supports it, and sometimes we don't—which is usually the case when we start to work this process. For instance, we may notice that we tend to become very defensive in conversations. What we may not realize is that we are defensive because we feel guilty and that we're trying to project the guilt away by blaming others. Once we recognize that we carry a lot of guilt, we can ask what the belief is that we hold that supports the guilt and the conditioning that created this belief. In this case, it could be a belief that we should be punished, one that came from our parents because we were punished without good reason. Or we may see that we constantly try to control others or situations, but it could take some time to realize that this way of operating comes from fear which originated in childhood when we didn't experience feeling safe. Even if we don't immediately know the belief and conditioning, they will be revealed to us at some point if we are committed to the process of healing. In general, we don't want to dwell on this second step or any step for too long— *unless* recognition of something brings up a strong emotional reaction—like experiencing grief over parents who were not there for us, to cite the examples above. Then let the tears and the process flow until its natural conclusion. In the early stages of becoming more aware of our unhealthy emotional patterns, as we initially work on new awarenesses, we may feel a lot of strong emotions like anger, grief, fear, shame, or guilt. After we have worked with a particular issue for some time, we can often move through the cycle quickly, since we've done a lot of the foundational healing work.

The third step in the cycle is to have compassion for ourselves—which may also have a forgiveness component—as well as for those who were responsible for the conditioning, if that's what comes up for us. Exercising compassion is an extremely important step that can actually be initiated at any point, especially if we tend to fall back into self-judgment, as most of us do. Anytime we feel that we are judging ourselves for any reason, we can immediately go to self-compassion. Recognize that judgment of others is a projection of judgment of ourselves, and go to compassion.

The fourth step is acceptance that this unhealed paradigm is where you currently are *but* that also this reality is something you'd like to change—and here we see the paradox again. Acceptance doesn't mean accepting that the belief is true. For instance, if we believe that we are lazy because we are not being productive or working all of the time, we are not necessarily accepting this belief as true. It could be true in that we may truly be a lazy and unmotivated person who is not being productive. Or it could be that we have been conditioned to believe that not working all of the time means we are lazy, and in this case, we're just accepting that we have this false belief about ourselves that we can't fully release yet. There are many layers of "reality," and this is why self-analysis is critical.

The fifth step, which Jesus demonstrated so well, is kenosis, or self-emptying. This step acknowledges our true state of being in unity with God, for we are clear vessels, but we also have blockages from our collective and individual humanity that we are healing and need to release. We want to be present in our bodies and envision and feel ourselves as a hollow tube or reed through which God and universal energy flow unobstructed.

The last step in the cycle is gratitude—gratitude that we are growing in awareness of our unity and of what we need to let go of that doesn't serve us.

We can do the healing cycle many times a day as we witness our thoughts, and when we have a strong reaction to something, and once we know the steps, the process becomes automatic because it is innate to us. Within a short time, there will be some parts that we don't have to consciously undertake. For instance, I no longer have to consciously orient myself in a place of self-compassion when self-judgment arises because it is now ingrained in me, but I still often go to compassion as the first step because it is so powerful. Or I may go immediately to the self-emptying stage, since energetically I can feel that something is off and this step helps to clear it, regardless of what it specifically relates to. Often, I hold the self-emptying for many minutes, which acknowledges the power of God as the healing force. There is not a perfect or right way to do the healing cycle, and as you continue to use it, it will take slightly different forms. Your intention to heal and go through the steps are as important as the steps themselves.

We are not ultimately in control of whether we have a physical cure for cancer. Again, how we define a "cure" is relative, but I am using the word in the sense of how the medical establishment and society define it—cancer that is in remission and doesn't show up on diagnostics. What we can control is the inputs that we give ourselves so that we have the best chance to heal at all levels, including through a physical cure. These holistic investments in our healing could possibly include conventional treatments to changes in our stress levels through changes in diet, lifestyle, and other factors, and especially to changes in our belief systems and emotional and spiritual constitutions and foundations through something like the healing cycle.

There are two levels of inputs or actions we can take, and they can be viewed as works and faith. One is the physical actions, or works—treatment, diet, lifestyle, meditation, yoga, or getting in nature, among other examples—and the other is what is happening with us internally, like how we deal with the fear, how we process our emotions and clear what is false in us, how we are strengthened or possibly weakened in our faith, and how we surrender, which is a definition of faith. If we are not reacting from fear but are instead spending the time to sift through and sit with information, this process will be an important bridge between our faith and potential physical actions. If we are doing this properly, it forces us to be patient and not to make a rushed decision but rather to feel into what is right for us.

We need to find a balance within and between the two types of actions—one that is *right for us*. For instance, when it comes to the physical actions we choose to take, as we have discussed, we need to throw a lot of things at the wall to give ourselves the best chance. But we also don't want to be in fear and think we have to do everything under the sun. Doing so will stress us out and be counterproductive. With the internal set of actions, the surrender part is super important, since again, we are not in control, and we need to accept that. Surrendering can be difficult for many individuals who are accustomed to controlling their environments, relationships, and careers; this is why I used the example above of not feeling safe if we are not in control. Many of these individuals are high achievers, and it's not an accident that these people get cancer because they haven't paid attention to the stressful and often unbalanced lives they are living—not to mention the tremendous amount of energy it takes and the stress of trying to control others and life itself. We are meant to live our lives in balance, and the universe is always pointing us there.

We are Spirit existing in this Earth reality as a temporary individual point of consciousness. We each have amazing gifts that are unique to us, gifts that we are meant to share with the world, and we are here to remember our divinity and awaken to who we truly are so that we can use these gifts. Unless we have risen to the consciousness of a high spiritual master like Jesus, death of the body is inevitable. But it does not need to be feared as so many do. Every moment here in a physical body is precious and holy, and then we leave this reality and return to a much larger reality that we know well.

Receiving a physical curing of your cancer *has no bearing on what you came here to achieve.* You can come into an awareness of your divinity and higher self with or without a physical cure. But as we have seen with others who have experienced terminal illnesses, the illness and the recognition that those who face them will die soon can be a powerful vehicle which thrusts someone out of their egoic thinking mind and into a much higher awareness—and many have also come to this realization on their deathbeds. This is the concept of death before death, what Jesus was referring to when he said we need to be born again.

This is true healing—healing of the mind and spirit, regardless of the final outcome for the physical body. If you have cancer, use it for the highest purpose. If your loved one has cancer, you can also use it for the highest purpose for you to face your fears. Again, everything in life can be manna—an amazing spiritual gift—for us. If we walk through life with this recognition, we will begin to see this truth in the smallest of things and experiences. So, in the grand scheme of things, if we apply a high understanding and we surrender, we will be at peace with whatever the outcome of our cancer treatment may be, and we will achieve what we came here to do. This doesn't mean that part of us, the human part who is cared for and loved by others, doesn't want to stay here. I want to stay here and grow old with my wife and see my grandchildren grow up. There is much left that I want to do and that God needs me to do, and I assume that I would take appropriate actions to do that, which may include further treatment if needed. But I don't know that for certain, since I am here right now, addressing what is in front of me without placing myself in future scenarios. That's all any of us can do, and that is the only place peace can be found.

FALSE BELIEF

NUMBER EIGHTEEN

> *I AM DAMAGED GOODS*

A S WE HAVE DISCUSSED, THE MIND IS VERY POWERFUL, especially when it is operating from false beliefs that we have about ourselves and of which we may not yet be aware. In addition, many of these beliefs are reinforced by entrenched societal conditioning. Even if we know that we are whole and complete within God, we still exist in a human body, which in some way we may consider damaged when we have been through a major health illness. For some reason, this seems especially true with cancer, likely because there is such a negative connotation around that label.

I realized this was the case for me *as I wrote this book*. I had finished treatment but was still needing to do a CT scan three months after treatment to confirm there was no sign of cancer. With the exceptions that I have noted, everything I have written in this book has been part of my direct experience or has come from God and the deepest part of my being, especially the parts about understanding our wholeness and perfection. Yet, at some level, I still had a partial belief that I was damaged goods, a belief I needed to work through. Logically—and I am grateful that I have that strong logical mind—I know this makes no sense. As I discussed in the preface—because it was obviously one of the most important points to make—we all have cancer to some degree. So, at a minimum, after my treatment and the other substantial changes I made, I have "less" cancer to some degree, right? I likely have much "less" than when I started, again depending on how it is labeled. But as we know, this is all relative. I am in better health than maybe I have been in a very long time—maybe in my whole life—because I ate very poorly for the first half of my life. Thus, the question becomes *Why would I think of myself as damaged goods?*

What pops in my head—what's usually a good pointer to lead us to a false belief within us—is how a car is listed as damaged on the Carfax-style report when it has been in an accident or had water damage. Its history follows it forever. I guess our history follows us forever, too, but we aren't cars, and someone can't look at us and know our history.

I believe that a part of me felt that I was damaged goods because I was the last person who I thought would have gotten cancer. There are several false beliefs—*unique to me*—that may be wrapped up in this illusion, from thinking I was doing most of the right things for my health to spiritual pride. The fact that this false belief about being damaged was coming up meant that I was still dealing with the aftereffects of the cancer journey post-treatment. I had not fully moved on, but none of us should move on until we have allowed the vehicle of cancer to serve us in all of the ways it needs to. I am extremely grateful for the continued awareness and release of false beliefs within me.

When we recognize that we are being led by a loving God and universe to become aware of our false beliefs and what isn't serving our highest good, we find ourselves in a great state of self-compassion, and we also have great compassion for others, since everybody is in the same boat. Compassion places us in the heart of God.

Sometimes life doesn't seem fair, like when we get cancer despite doing everything "right," or when there doesn't seem to be justice in the world—why does it seem like this "bad" person or group is being rewarded? But we don't understand how fairness and justice should be defined, which brings us back to the restrictive nature of labels. We are applying *our* black-and-white and inflexible judgment system to a universe that is not based on separation and distinctions. It is a waste of time to continue asking why. It is not a waste of time to temporarily look back and ask *how*—how did I get to this point where I developed active cancer so that I can now change my health going forward? But many things in the universe remain a mystery and are meant to be that way. The sooner we accept that reality, the sooner we can be at peace. As we increasingly trust more in God and the universe that if we just pay attention to what life is showing us—trusting that our highest good will be done—we will reach a point where we know God to be actively working in our lives at all times. Eventually our trust becomes complete and we no longer have the need to ask any questions.

Each of us is holy, pure, perfect, and whole because of our divinity. So, none of us are damaged goods after a serious health issue, relationship dissolution, or job layoff, for example. We have to stop applying our judgments to these situations—especially applying them to ourselves—and just see these "adverse" events as part of a vast continuum of life. Think about it this way. What is the difference between these two statements? I see the world as it is, and the world is as I see it? With the latter we are seeing the world and our place in it through our own unique colored lens. With the former we have taken off our colored glasses and we just see what exists when judgment is not applied to a situation or person. And that is heaven.

AFTERWORD

UNFORTUNATELY, DURING THE MONTHS IT TOOK TO WRITE AND edit this book, I learned of a number of others—a family member, friends, and acquaintances—who were diagnosed with cancer. Some of their prognoses are good; some are not so good. As I have spoken to these individuals or their spouses, my heart has both opened and broken for them, because I know the fear that accompanies cancer or any major health issue. I want to take away their fear and pain, because we are not meant to live in suffering. This is not what God intended for this world. But we have to deal with reality, and sometimes that means that life will bring us difficult circumstances.

Many years of working on myself and being in observation of others have increasingly brought me to the understanding that we can't figure things out—that there are no absolutes in life, no blacks and whites, and certainly no guarantees one way or the other. For instance, two years prior to my cancer diagnosis I had a full blood work test done, and my doctor said that my blood work reflected perfect health. He said to keep doing what I was doing. I was fortunate to be able to catch my cancer because I was able to physically feel it. If I hadn't been able to do that, it may have been at a much later stage when I first became aware of it, which is the situation for so many. This is the reason we all need to examine our lives and address the areas we have discussed in this book—now—whether we have "cancer" or not.

Accepting the mystery of life takes us to a place of surrender in awe and in wonder and gratitude. We can then apply this practice of faith—and its ups and downs— to the cancer journey, which is integral to healing in the complete way.

I have great trust in each of you who is undergoing a cancer or a significant health issue journey. I believe that each of you has the strength to look within and find your answers and your balance, for a middle-of-the-road, balanced approach is always the wisest. I know with complete certainty that you can tap into your divinity and innate wisdom and change your life in the most amazing way. That you can truly make the best of a difficult situation. What I hope and pray for is that you will know this yourself with complete certainty and take the steps that are revealed to you and will be highly beneficial for you. But I have also observed human behavior long enough to know that a majority of people who read this book—likely a large majority— will not examine their lives to any depth. Unfortunately, they will not take significant steps to any large degree and will find themselves in the same place, in the same ruts, and going around the same circles they have always been. It is really true that one definition of insanity is doing the same thing and expecting different results.

Everyone gets to make the choices they want to make, but each of us needs to realize that every choice or non-choice has consequences. I have compassion for those who cannot make significant changes in their lives, because intuitively we know that change can create pain and we shy away from that, usually fooling ourselves with some type of justification or rationalization. This is human nature. But God can only help us with healing in the complete way and can help us see the gifts in our illness to the extent we are willing to help ourselves. If we are aware and blessed enough to see that we cannot and will not make significant changes, we can move into self-compassion, which is a choice that has highly beneficial consequences.

Whatever we choose, it is important to recognize how easily we fall into self-judgment and think that we have failed, that we are not doing something right, or that we have let someone down if we choose a certain path of treatment. Here we can see the way our minds and conditioning take us down a path that is not beneficial. Again, we can and must always come back to observation and self-compassion. We can make the recognition that cancer sucks while also holding the recognition that it is a wake-up call that can be a gift for us.

This book was written and revised over a number of months. The growth that I went through with my cancer journey, which included the writing of this book, has pushed me to an even higher awareness in many areas, and for that I am highly grateful. Interestingly, I wrote earlier in the book that I chose to have conventional treatment because I did not feel at that time that I could heal it on my own. I feel this might be different if I were having to make that decision again today. But usually it is the very vehicle—in this case my cancer journey—that enables us to have a higher understanding where we can look back and say that we would have done it differently. Life has so many interesting threads and nuances.

I have now had several follow-up CT scans every three

months. Thankfully, the scans have shown that I am now likely "cancer-free." The waiting was somewhat easy the first two months between scans, since I couldn't do anything to find out the effectiveness of the treatment, so I was able to put it out of my mind and just do life. But as the date approached for each scan, I became increasingly fearful. I was looking outside of myself for an outcome that I wanted, and all I could do was fall back into self-compassion. It's important to recognize that we are both human and divine, so we are going to feel fear and other "negative" emotions, but we have our divine toolbox to help us process and transform these negative emotions.

Each time I found out the results of the scan, my first emotion besides relief was gratitude and an extreme appreciation for being on this earth with my family. Life is a gift, and it should not be taken for granted. Most of us are frantically running around trying to achieve something, and we miss the simplicity and beauty of life, especially the joy found in our relationships with those we love and in our connection to the natural world. We are really here on Earth for communion. Having a journey with cancer or another severe health issue will hopefully awaken us to what's important. Otherwise, the experience will be wasted if no greater awareness and love comes out of it.

I wish you the greatest of blessings and comfort on your healing journey. We are one family, and we all need each other.

With gratitude and love,
Larry

If this book has provided benefit for you, I would
greatly appreciate your leaving an online review.
I love to communicate with readers,
so please visit my website at

www.lawrencedoochin.com